Contents

KU-014-733

Preface to the first edition   vii

Preface to the second edition   viii

Part I   General principles   1

1 Historical introduction   3

2 Pharmacology of central nervous system transmission   9

3 Factors influencing the action of psychotropic drugs   35

4 Methods of studying behavioural effects of drugs   48

5 Social and psychological aspects of drug treatment   71

Part II   Clinical applications   85

6 Schizophrenia   87

7 Affective disorders   120

8 Anxiety   149

9 Organic psychiatric syndromes   166

10 Personality disorders, alcoholism and drug dependence   174

11 Sleep disturbance   191

12 Sexual problems   203

13 Disorders of appetite and body weight   214

14 Pain   229

15 Child psychiatry   238

16 The management of overdosage of centrally acting drugs   245

Subject index   251

Index of drug names   262

Figures and tables

Figures

1 The distribution of noradrenergic and dopaminergic
pathways in the brain   12
2 Diagrammatic representation of a central monoaminergic
synapse showing possible sites of drug action   24
3 Number of prescriptions issued by general practitioners
for 'tranquillisers' in England and Wales, 1961–73   72
4 The neurochemical feedback loop in the nigrostriatal
system   97
5 The metabolic pathways of chlorpromazine   98
6 The metabolic pathways of the benzodiazepines   154
7 Diagram to illustrate role of substantia gelatinosa in
acting as a gate-control system in regulating input of
sensory information into the central nervous pathways
concerned with the perception of, and response to, pain   231

Tables

1 Classification of sympathomimetic amines into
predominant direct and indirect activity   28
2 Clinically important interactions involving psychotropic
drugs   44
3 Effect of research design on the outcome of clinical trials   65
4 Effect of statistical analysis on the outcome of clinical
trials   68
5 Percentage of the adult population who had taken
anxiolytic sedative drugs in the previous twelve months   73
6 Neuroleptic drugs   111
7 Antidepressant drugs   140
8 Anxiolytic drugs   162
9 Hypnotics   200

Drug treatment
in psychiatry

Social and Psychological Aspects of Medical Practice

Editor: Trevor Silverstone

Also in this series:

Malcolm Lader
The Psychophysiology of Mental Illness

J. Stuart Whiteley and John Gordon
Group Approaches in Psychiatry

Drug treatment in psychiatry

Trevor Silverstone, MA, DM, FRCP, FRCPsych, DPM
Reader in Human Psychopharmacology
and Consultant Psychiatrist,
St Bartholomew's Hospital, London

Paul Turner, MD, BSc, FRCP
Professor of Clinical Pharmacology,
St Bartholomew's Hospital, London

Routledge & Kegan Paul
London, Henley and Boston

First published in 1974
Second edition 1978
by Routledge & Kegan Paul Ltd
39 Store Street,
London WC1E 7DD,
Broadway House,
Newtown Road,
Henley-on-Thames,
Oxon RG9 1EN and
9 Park Street,
Boston, Mass. 02108, USA
Set in Monotype Imprint Series 101
by HBM Typesetting Ltd Standish Street Chorley Lancs
and printed in Great Britain by
Lowe & Brydone Ltd

British Library Cataloguing in Publication Data

Silverstone, Trevor
Drug treatment in psychiatry. – 2nd ed. –
(Social and psychological aspects of medical
practice).
1. Psychopharmacology   2. Mentally ill –
Care and treatment
I. Title   II. Series   III. Turner, Paul
616.8'918   RC483   78-40127

ISBN 0 7100 8933 3
ISBN 0 7100 8934 1   Pbk

Preface to the first edition

This book was written to provide an introduction to psycho-pharmacology for all those who are concerned in the management of psychiatric disorders, whether in the community or in hospital.

We have attempted to place drug therapy on a sound physio-logical and pharmacological basis wherever possible. To this end we begin each clinical section by reviewing what is known of the underlying physiological and biochemical factors in the condition under consideration; we then proceed to discuss the pharmacology of the various drugs used in its treatment before going on to outline a recommended course of treatment. At the end of the chapters on schizophrenia, affective disorders, anxiety and sleep a list of relev-ant drugs is given together with doses and, where appropriate, our comments.

The form of presentation which we have chosen has led to some repetition; we consider this a small price to pay for a compre-hensive discussion of a particular clinical condition, or group of conditions, within a single chapter. Rather than giving detailed references within the text, at the end of each chapter we have recommended suitable sources of further information.

We express our gratitude to Professor Linford Rees and to Professor Sir Eric Scowen for providing us with the opportunities for pursuing our interests in the field of clinical psychopharma-cology. We also thank Mrs Gail Frampton for all the secretarial assistance she has given us.

TS and PT

Preface to the second edition

We are naturally most gratified that the response to the first edition of this book was such that a second edition has been called for so soon. This has given us an opportunity to make some editorial changes, as well as to update the contents, although the basic aims, as set out in the preface to the first edition, remain the same.

The suggestions for further reading, given at the end of each chapter, have been considerably enlarged; this will, we trust, allow the interested reader to delve more easily into the relevant scientific literature. We have added one new chapter, chapter 3, which covers the subjects of pharmacokinetics and drug inter-action. The section on the management of overdosage of centrally acting drugs, which was an appendix in the first edition, has now been promoted to chapter status (chapter 16).

Helpful suggestions concerning the revision of our book have come from a large number of people, and to them we convey our thanks. In addition certain colleagues have most kindly responded to our request for their views and comments on particular chapters; these include: Dr Constance Dennehy (child psychiatry), Dr Allan Gardner (organic psychiatric syndromes), Dr Jill Fincham (methods of studying behavioural effects of drugs), Dr John Reed and Dr John Mack (drug dependence); to them our especial gratitude.

As before, Mrs Gail Frampton has provided a most efficient secretarial service with great forbearing, for which we thank her warmly.

TS and PT

General principles

Part I

Historical introduction

A desire to take medicine is, perhaps, the great feature which distinguishes man from other animals.

William Osler, 1894

A drug, according to the World Health Organisation, is 'any substance which when taken into the living organism may modify one of its functions'. Psychotropic drugs are those which have, through their action on the brain, an effect on normal and abnormal psychological processes.

Perhaps the first such substance to be discovered, certainly the first to be referred to in Western literature, is alcohol: 'and Noah began to be a husbandman, and he planted a vineyard and he drank of the wine, and was drunken . . . .' In fact it is unlikely that there ever was a time when alcoholic beverages were not used; certainly the Egyptians drank freely of them and there is a picture dating from 1500 B.C. illustrating the unfortunate effects of drinking to excess. The word itself stems from the Arabic *al kihl* meaning essence, and *alcohol vini* referred to the essential or most subtle part of the wine.

Several other substances which are both used and abused in present-day society have almost as extended a lineage as has alcohol. Opium poppy seeds have been discovered in Stone Age settlements in Switzerland dating from at least 2000 B.C. Homer described the action of nepenthe, which most authorities believe to be synonymous with opium, as giving 'forgetfulness of evil'. There is even some suggestion that the secret of opium, probably coming from Egypt, was closely guarded by the élite and was given to certain chosen warriors (heroes) before such epic battles as Troy. The habit of taking opium spread throughout Europe and the East in spite of warnings against intemperate use; until de Quincey, in the early nineteenth century, vividly

3

portrayed the agonies which could come from dependence on it, most Englishmen regarded opium as but a simple family remedy.

Another drug which acts on the central nervous system, known to the ancients and still with us, is marihuana, the derivative of *Cannabis indica*. A Chinese emperor writing in 2200 B.C. referred to its euphoric properties and advised that its use should be restricted, as in his opinion it was little more than a 'liberator of sin'. Perhaps the most famous users of marihuana, or hashish, were the assassins (whose very name derived from the word hashish), a fanatical thirteenth-century Persian sect who, when intoxicated, would recklessly commit the most brutal murders.

On the other side of the world, in South America, the leaf of the coca tree containing cocaine, was until quite recently as widely taken by the indigenous peoples of the Andes as alcohol in our society. Unlike alcohol, which is a sedative, cocaine is a central stimulant and allowed the Incas and their descendants to work prodigiously without fatigue. Because of this property its use was encouraged by the Spanish mine-owners.

Even stranger are the effects of *peyotl*, the sacred cactus of Mexico. This contains mescaline, a potent hallucinogenic compound, which so distorts the processes of perception that brilliant dream-like visions may be experienced. More recently other hallucinogenic substances such as lysergic acid diethylamide (LSD) have enjoyed a certain vogue and have even been employed to some extent in psychiatric treatment, although with doubtful effect.

The drugs thus far considered have all been taken in the first instance to obtain a state of pleasurable relaxation or contentment; it was only much later that the isolation of the active principle of opium and morphine, in 1817, and of cocaine in 1885, allowed a medicinal application.

An ancient remedy from India, *Rauwolfia serpentina*, which has always been used therapeutically rather than socially, turned out to be of considerable theoretical and practical interest. Indian texts have for three thousand years recommended the root of this plant, which contains reserpine, in cases of psychiatric disturbance, a recommendation which was found in the 1950s to be soundly based, and reserpine was among the first of the newer 'tranquillising' drugs (see chapter 6).

In 1952, the same year as reserpine was formally introduced into modern psychiatry, Delay and Deniker described the dramatic

4

effect of the wholly synthetic compound chlorpromazine (Largactil, Thaorzine) in cases of schizophrenia, and in so doing may be said to have inaugurated the sub-specialty of psychopharmacology which has grown so rapidly in the past two decades. As with many other important therapeutic advances, the use of chlorpromazine was based on a chance observation. Promethazine, an antihistamine drug, was noted to exhibit sedative effects, and chlorpromazine, which is chemically related to promethazine (they are both phenothiazines), was synthesised in the hope of increasing this sedative action. However, it was found that its range of activity was much wider, and it was soon being prescribed for a variety of conditions, particularly schizophrenia and mania.

Shortly after the synthesis and clinical investigation of chlorpromazine another breakthrough came with the discovery of the monoamine oxidase inhibitors. As in the case of chlorpromazine, this also arose out of an unexpected clinical observation, namely that tuberculous patients being treated with iproniazid became rather more euphoric than might have been expected. As a result it was suggested that if iproniazid did have a real mood-elevating action, it might be related to its ability to inhibit the enzyme monoamine oxidase, and thereby affect brain amine concentrations (see chapter 2). If this were so it was further reasoned that such compounds might be of considerable therapeutic benefit in cases of depression. Although iproniazid itself was soon found to be too toxic for widespread application, a variety of other less toxic monoamine oxidase inhibitors have been synthesised, and the introduction of this class of drugs has greatly stimulated investigation into the biochemical basis of depression itself (see chapter 7).

As frequently happens, the discovery of one major new drug like chlorpromazine leads to a hurried search for other members of the same chemical class which, it is hoped, will prove more effective than the original compound. In the course of such a search, drugs bearing a superficial structural resemblance to the parent compound may be found to cause clinical effects quite different from those expected. Such was the case with imipramine (Tofranil), which was originally synthesised in the hope of producing an iminodibenzyl derivative related to chlorpromazine with an even stronger sedative action. On clinical trial imipramine had little sedative activity but did exhibit a marked antidepressant activity—a property which had not been forecast. Since then many

5

other drugs in the same group (the tricyclic antidepressants) have been introduced (see chapter 7).

Among the more significant advances to have taken place in recent years has been the confirmation of Cade's earlier report that the element lithium is effective in improving the symptoms of mania. Not only does lithium relieve the acute symptoms, it appears to have a true prophylactic activity in preventing recurrences of both the manic and depressive episodes which occur in those patients who are predisposed to manic-depressive psychosis (see chapter 7).

The newer synthetic drugs thus far considered, the phenothiazines, the monoamine oxidase inhibitors and the tricyclic antidepressants, have all been directed mainly at the more severe forms of psychiatric illness, the psychoses. There remains, however, a great deal of minor psychological distress, mainly manifested as anxiety or the somatic accompaniments of anxiety, which accounts for a considerable proportion of the conditions presenting in general practice and internal medicine. Therefore any drug that can relieve such anxiety symptoms will obviously have a ready appeal. The barbiturates, the first of which, malonylurea (barbituric acid, possibly named in honour of St Barbara), was synthesised in 1864, are still considered by some to be the most effective, and certainly the cheapest, antianxiety compounds. There is, however, a considerable danger of drug dependence developing (see chapter 10) and other anxiolytic drugs have recently been introduced which are claimed to be less addictive and less sedating. Among the first was meprobamate (Equanil, Miltown) which swept the USA in the 1950s. It has, however, been largely superseded by the benzodiazepines chlordiazepoxide and diazepam which, according to one authority, have been prescribed in the past five years to more patients throughout the world than any other single compound.

Since the 1950s when most of the drugs discussed were originally introduced, largely, as we have seen, due to chance, there has been a spate of new variants. There are currently available at least twenty-eight phenothiazine derivatives, seventeen antidepressants of the monoamine reuptake inhibitor type, nine monoamine oxidase inhibitors, and twenty-five non-barbiturate sedatives and hypnotics. Not only the variety, but also the total number, of prescriptions for these drugs are rising rapidly.

Furthermore, it has become almost impossible to keep up with the enormous volume of published material pouring out each year.

In 1969 the number of papers written on psychopharmacology alone was over 3,500 and the USA Government has considered it necessary to create a special department within its National Institute of Mental Health to cope with the monumental task of coding and indexing this flood of papers.

In a welcome attempt to provide some shape and order to this welter of information, and to assist the study of psychopharmacology generally, a committee of the World Health Organisation suggested the following classification of psychotropic drugs.

1 *Neuroleptics:* drugs with therapeutic effects on psychoses and other types of psychiatric disorder. In addition they usually produce extrapyramidal effects, such as tremor and rigidity.
(a) Phenothiazines: e.g. chlorpromazine (Largactil, Thorazine)
(b) Thioxanthenes: e.g. thiothixene (Navane)
(c) Butyrophenones: e.g. haloperidol (Serenace, Haldol)
(d) Diphenylbutylpiperidines: e.g. pimozide (Orap)
(e) Reserpine derivatives

2 *Anxiolytic sedatives:* substances that reduce pathological anxiety, tension and agitation, without therapeutic effect on disturbed cognitive or perceptual processes. These drugs usually raise the convulsive threshold and do not produce extrapyramidal or autonomic effects. They may produce drug dependence.
(a) Propanediols: e.g. meprobamate (Equanil, Miltown)
(b) Benzodiazepines: e.g. diazepam (Valium)
(c) Barbiturates: e.g. amylobarbitone sodium (Sodium Amytal)

3 *Antidepressants:* drugs effective in the treatment of pathological depressive states.
(a) Monoamine oxidase inhibitors: e.g. phenelzine (Nardil)
(b) Monoamine reuptake inhibitors: e.g. imipramine (Tofranil)

4 *Psychostimulants:* drugs that increase the level of alertness and/ or motivation.
(a) Amphetamines: e.g. dexamphetamine (Dexedrine)
(b) Caffeine

5 *Psychodysleptics:* drugs producing abnormal mental phenomena, particularly in the cognitive and perceptual spheres.
(a) Lysergic acid diethylamide
(b) Mescaline
(c) Psylocybin

(d) Dimethyltryptophan
(e) Cannabis

The above classification will be used throughout this book. The compounds are discussed in association with the various conditions covered. Each chapter consists of an introduction to the underlying physiology and pathology of the given conditions (as far as they are known); this is followed by a discussion of the pharmacology of the various drugs used in their treatment; in the final section a recommended therapeutic approach, using the drugs already discussed, is presented.

Suggestions for further reading

AYD, F., and BLACKWELL, B., *Discoveries in Biological Psychiatry*, Lippincott, Philadelphia, 1970.

INGLIS, B., *The Forbidden Game, A Social History of Drugs*, Hodder & Stoughton, London, 1975.

JOHNSON, F. N., and CADE, J. F. J., 'The historical background to lithium research and therapy', in *Lithium Research and Therapy*, ed. F. N. Johnson, Academic Press, London, 1975.

LEWIN, L., *Phantastica—Narcotic and Stimulating Drugs, Their Use and Abuse*, Routledge & Kegan Paul, London, 1931 (reprinted 1964).

SWAZEY, J. P., *Chlorpromazine in Psychiatry, A Study of Therapeutic Innovation*, MIT Press, Cambridge, Mass., 1974.

WORLD HEALTH ORGANISATION, *Research in Psychopharmacology*, WHO Technical Report, series no. 371, 1967.

Pharmacology of central nervous system transmission 2

Neurohumoral transmission

The effects of drugs on mood, perception and consciousness can best be understood in terms of their actions on the underlying chemical mechanisms responsible for normal function of the central nervous system.

The contacts between one nerve cell and another within the central nervous system as well as in the peripheral autonomic ganglia are called 'synapses'. This term was first introduced by Sherrington in 1897 and is derived from the Greek word *synopsis*, meaning 'clasp'. It reflects the intimate nature of the contact between cells, which Sherrington, like others before him, recognised to be present.

The mechanism by which nerve impulses are propagated from one cell across the synapse to the other was a matter of considerable controversy until the middle of this century. According to one school of thought, synaptic transmission could be explained solely in terms of electrical events, whereas a second school of thought maintained that nerve impulses were transmitted by chemical substances released from the nerve endings. This idea was strengthened at the turn of the century by the observations of Lewandowsky and Langley that injection of extracts from adrenal glands produced similar effects in experimental animals to stimulation of sympathetic nerves. Elliott, in 1904, suggested that sympathetic nerve impulses released minute amounts of an adrenaline-like substance in close contact with the effector cells. In 1907, Dixon drew attention to the close similarity between the effects of the alkaloid muscarine and responses to vagal stimulation, and put forward the hypothesis that such stimulation liberated a muscarine-like substance, which acted as a chemical transmitter of the impulses to the effector cell. It was not until 1921, however, that Loewi demonstrated that stimulation of the vagus nerve of one frog heart released a

9

substance into the perfusion fluid which slowed the rate of a second heart when the perfusion fluid flowed through it. Loewi and Navratil went on to show that this substance was acetylcholine.

It is now generally agreed that transmission at most, if not all, synapses in the mammalian central nervous system is mediated by chemical agents. These are released by action potentials which pass down the axon, and interact with receptors on the post-synaptic effector cell body to increase its permeability to ions and set up a further action potential within it.

Before a compound can be considered to be a neurochemical transmitter it should conform to the following criteria:

1 it must be present in the nerve endings
2 the neurone must contain the enzymes necessary for its manu-facture and release
3 the presence of various precursors in the synthetic pathway should be demonstrable
4 there should be systems for the inactivation of the transmitter; where enzymes are involved, they should be demonstrable within the neurone or in its immediate vicinity
5 during nerve stimulation the substance should be detectable in extracellular fluid collected from the region of the activated synapses
6 when applied to the post-synaptic cell body the substance should mimic the action of the synaptically released transmitter
7 drugs which are thought to produce their effect by interaction within the transmitter should be shown to interact with it in the predicted manner under experimental conditions.

The last two criteria are probably the most important.

The bodies of nerve cells in the central nervous system are densely covered by synapses, and it is probable that they have more than one transmitter substance acting on their surfaces. It has been shown, for example, that at least three transmitters act on one type of cell, the Renshaw cell in the spinal cord, two of them being excitatory transmitters and one an inhibitory transmitter. Other experiments have shown that neurones in the cerebral cortex are inhibited by at least two distinct transmitter substances.

When it is recalled how difficult it was to demonstrate neuro-humoral transmission in relatively simple peripheral synapses, and that it is only in recent years that all the seven criteria listed above have been satisfied for them, the difficulties of unequivocally demonstrating transmitter substances in the central nervous system will be appreciated. In fact, the evidence for most of the substances which have been postulated to act in the central nervous system is only circumstantial and fulfils but a few of these criteria.

Among the numerous substances thus far suggested the most important are:

acetylcholine
adrenaline
noradrenaline
dopamine
5-hydroxytryptamine (serotonin)
histamine
l-glutamic acid
gamma-aminobutyric acid (GABA)
prostaglandins
substance P

Acetylcholine

Acetylcholine together with appropriate enzymes for its synthesis and degradation is present in the central nervous system. Histochemical studies have revealed probable cholinergic pathways to the cerebral cortex in the ascending reticular system and in the cerebellum. Microinjection techniques using iontophoresis have shown that neurones sensitive to acetylcholine are present in all regions of the central nervous system. In the spinal cord acetylcholine produces only excitation of neuronal activity, but in other parts of the central nervous system and brain both excitatory and inhibitory effects may be seen. The effects of acetylcholine in the spinal cord seem to be mainly nicotinic, while those in the cerebral cortex are predominantly muscarinic and can be blocked by antimuscarinic agents such as atropine and hyoscine. The central effects of these drugs differ, atropine having excitant and hyoscine depressant actions, and they probably depend on their anticholinergic effects on different groups of neurones in the brain.

Adrenaline (Epinephrine)

There is evidence that a neuronal system exists in the hypothalamic nuclei concerned with autonomic control in which adrenaline is the neurotransmitter. It has been suggested that this is a vasodepressor system, and that the antihypertensive effects of clonidine

may depend on direct activation of adrenergic rather than noradrenergic receptors. If this is so, then chlorpromazine and
haloperidol should be adrenaline-receptor blocking drugs since
they antagonise clonidine-induced hypotension in experimental
animals.

Noradrenaline (norepinephrine)

Noradrenaline, unlike acetylcholine, is not widely distributed
throughout the central nervous system, but is concentrated in the
hypothalamus and brain stem (see Figure 1). Fluorescent histochemical techniques have shown specific neuronal pathways which
form and store noradrenaline; these are particularly localised in the
hypothalamus. Such fibres fluoresce with an intense green colour.
There is a marked similarity between noradrenaline-containing
neurones in the brain and those in the peripheral sympathetic

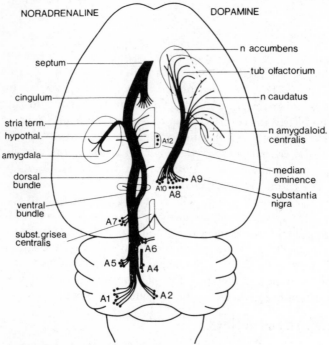

Horizontal projection of the ascending NA and DA pathways.

Figure 1 *The distribution of noradrenergic and dopaminergic pathways
in the brain* (after U. Ungerstedt, *Acta Physiologica Scandinavica
Supplement* no. 367, 1971)

nervous system. In both, noradrenaline is highly concentrated in the nerve terminals with much lower concentrations in other parts of the cell and the terminal regions of both types of cell are similar, showing much branching and varicosity.

Microinjection techniques have demonstrated that noradrenaline has an inhibitory action on the Renshaw cells in the spinal cord, which are excited by acetylcholine. In the cerebral cortex it depresses neuronal activity, while in the brain stem both excitation and inhibition occur. Bradley and Wolstencroft found in experimental animals that about 80 per cent of the nerve cells in the medulla and pons responded to applications of noradrenaline, 20 per cent showing excitation and 60 per cent inhibition. Chlorpromazine, an adrenergic receptor blocking drug, appears to antagonise the transmitter actions of noradrenaline at those synapses where it is excitatory.

Dopamine

Dopamine is a precursor in the synthetic pathway of noradrenaline:

Phenylalanine⟶ Tyrosine⟶ Dopa ⟶ Dopamine⟶ Noradrenaline

It is not surprising, therefore, that it should be present in the brain in about the same amount as noradrenaline. It does not have the same distribution, however, which may indicate that it has an independent action. Fluorescent studies have shown that dopamine is particularly localised in the caudate nucleus and neighbouring striatal areas, and its importance in this region has been emphasised by the demonstration that patients with Parkinson's disease have a reduced dopamine content of the basal ganglia (see Figure 1). Drugs such as reserpine and alpha-methyl dopa which produce monoamine depletion in the brain, and hence reduce the dopamine content of the basal ganglia, produce clinical features of parkinsonism as an effect of over-dosage. Treatment of patients with Parkinson's disease with dopamine, administered either orally or intravenously, proved unsuccessful because dopamine does not pass readily from the circulation into the brain. However, its precursor levodopa does pass into the brain, and is presumably converted into dopamine by the enzyme dopa decarboxylase present within the neurones. Wide clinical experience has confirmed its usefulness in controlling many of the features of Parkinson's disease, particularly the rigidity and difficulty in fine movement. However, levodopa may itself produce a large number of undesirable central nervous effects including involuntary dyskinetic movements, sleep disturbance and a variety of psychological changes such as severe depression; agitation, confusion, delirium, paranoia, hallucinations, delusions and psychosis have also been reported. The extent to which such behavioural effects are due to dopamine acting itself as a central transmitter, or to its role as a precursor in the synthesis of noradrenaline, is at present not known.

It is probable that the effects of dopamine in the basal ganglia are opposed by acetylcholine and other muscarinic agents. One such compound, tremorine, produces a parkinsonian-like tremor in experimental animals which can be abolished by atropine and atropine-like drugs. The effectiveness of many established drugs in the treatment of Parkinson's disease such as benzhexol (Artane) and orphenadrine (Disipal) may, therefore, be due to their ability to block the central effects of acetylcholine.

Dopamine is also a transmitter in three other neuronal systems: (a) the medullary pathway which is intimately involved with the vomiting centre; (b) the meso-limbic pathway, a disorder of which may be involved in schizophrenia; (c) the hypothalamic-pituitary pathway which controls the release of prolactin from the pituitary gland.

While levodopa increases dopamine activity indirectly after decarboxylation, drugs are now available which stimulate central dopamine receptors directly, including apomorphine, bromocriptine and piribedil. Apomorphine is a potent stimulator of receptors in the vomiting centre. Bromocriptine and piribedil are potent inhibitors of prolactin release, and also have some therapeutic value in Parkinson's disease. They produce nausea and vomiting in higher doses. The dose-related actions of these drugs to mediate these different effects suggest that a sub-classification of central dopamine receptors is now justified.

5-Hydroxytryptamine (Serotonin)

Like noradrenaline, 5-hydroxytryptamine (5HT) is concentrated mainly in the hypothalamus and brain stem. Neurones containing this monoamine show a yellow fluorescence in contrast to the green fluorescence of noradrenaline containing neurones. Tryptaminergic neurones are thought to extend from the brain stem up into the cerebral cortex and hippocampal areas. Microinjection studies have shown no effects of 5HT on nerve cells within the spinal cord, but in the cortex and brain stem it has both excitant and inhibitory actions, like noradrenaline. Of the cortical neurones which respond to application of 5HT, about 30 per cent are excited and 50 per cent inhibited. In the medulla and pons about 90 per cent of neurones respond, 40 per cent being excited and 50 per cent inhibited.

The possibility that 5HT is a central transmitter was suggested by the finding that the potent psychotomimetic hallucinogenic drug d-lysergic acid diethylamide (LSD) is a potent inhibitor of 5HT in peripheral tissues. It was tempting to suppose that its central effects, too, were due to 5HT antagonism, but against this hypothesis was the observation that the derivative of LSD, 2-bromolysergic acid diethylamide (BOL 148), which is as potent a 5HT antagonist as LSD, was devoid of psychotomimetic effects. More recent evidence, however, suggesting that methysergide and cinanserin, both potent 5HT antagonists in peripheral tissues, may be effective in controlling manic psychotic states (see chapter 6) adds weight to the suggestion that 5HT may have an important role in central transmission. It is of interest that the excitatory effects of 5HT in microinjection studies could be antagonised by LSD, BOL 148 and methysergide, while antagonism of its inhibitory effects was rare.

Responses of cells to more than one transmitter

Bradley and his collegues have studied with microinjection techniques the responses of cells in the brain and spinal cord to acetylcholine, noradrenaline and 5HT. In certain regions, such as the medulla, there were neurones which responded to all three substances; in some regions all the transmitters were excitatory, in others they were all inhibitory, and yet in others one compound might excite and the other two inhibit, or vice versa. In other regions of the brain more consistent patterns were observed, with all neurones responding in the same way to given transmitters, for example, acetylcholine and 5HT might have an excitatory action and noradrenaline might have an inhibitory action on all the neurones in the group. With such variations in response to the transmitter substances within the brain, it is not surprising that psychotropic drugs acting on these substances themselves show a wide diversity of effect.

Histamine

Histamine is present in the central nervous system together with its precursor histidine, in the same areas as noradrenaline and 5HT. Microinjection studies have shown that it depresses the excitatory threshold of many neurones in the spinal cord, and has both depressant and excitant effects on neurones in the cerebral cortex. Histidine, too, has a depressant action on cortical neurones.

The actions of histamine throughout the body appear to be mediated by two types of receptor, designated H_1 and H_2. The H_1 effects are contraction of smooth muscle of the intestine, bronchioles, uterus and large blood vessels, dilation of small blood vessels, especially venules, and increasing vascular permeability to plasma proteins. The most important H_2 receptor effect is stimulation of the acid-secreting cells in the gastric mucosa producing a profuse flow of gastric juice with a high acidity but relatively low pepsin content.

H_1 receptor antagonists such as mepyramine, chlorcyclizine and the other standard antihistamine drugs antagonise both the excitant and depressant actions of histamine on cortical neurones, but they also antagonise the depressant effects of acetylcholine, noradrenaline and 5HT. Thus the extent to which their central effects are due to antihistamine activity is uncertain.

H_2 receptors are selectively blocked by burimamide, metiamide and cimetidine. These drugs do not appear to have specific central nervous actions, and therefore it is not yet known whether there are H_2 receptors within the human brain.

L-Glutamic acid

L-glutamic acid and related amino acids such as aspartic, cysteic and homocysteic acids have excitant effects on nerve cells in many parts of the central nervous system. They are widely distributed throughout the brain and are released from the cerebral cortex during states of cortical activity. Evidence for the role of l-glutamic acid as a transmitter at invertebrate neuromuscular junctions has been established, and it may ultimately prove to have an important role in the human central nervous system.

Gamma-aminobutyric acid

Gamma-aminobutyric acid (GABA) is an amino acid, related structurally to glycine and taurine, which is restricted in its distribution in the body to the central nervous system. Unlike glutamic acid with its excitatory neuronal effects, GABA depresses activity of neurones in the spinal cord and brain. Animal studies have shown that it is released from the cerebral cortex in quantities which vary with the level of cortical activity, and some pharmacologists have suggested that GABA is, in fact, the main inhibitory transmitter in the cerebral cortex. Caution must be exercised in such studies, however, to exclude the possibility that the amino acids are derived from cerebrospinal fluid or non-neuronal elements rather than from nerve cells. Although the place of GABA in central transmission is still controversial, it may play a role in the pharmacological actions of benzodiazepine drugs (see chapter 8).

Prostaglandins

Prostaglandin was the name given by Von Euler in 1935 to a lipid substance derived from human seminal fluid which contracted smooth muscle. Substances with similar pharmacological activity were found in the seminal fluid of sheep, and in extracts of prostate and vesicular glands. Today the term 'prostaglandins' no longer refers to a single substance but to a large family of closely related long-chain unsaturated fatty acids, all derivatives of prostanoic acid.

Several prostaglandins are present in the mammalian central nervous system, and are released from the cerebral cortex into a perfusing fluid when peripheral nerves are stimulated. This release is depressed by drugs such as pentobarbitone and chlorpromazine. Some of these compounds have been studied with microinjection techniques and have excitant and inhibitory actions on various neurones in the brain stem. Their action is prolonged when compared with other transmitter substances such as acetylcholine and noradrenaline, and, although their presence in the brain and release on nerve stimulation suggests some function relating to transmission, it may be that this is more concerned with control or modulation of transmitter release or neuronal excitability than actual transmission. It may be relevant to this hypothesis that some

17

prostaglandins are released from phrenic nerve diaphragm preparations and from parasympathetic and sympathetic nerve endings during nerve stimulation, and it has been suggested that they may be part of a 'feedback' system regulating transmitter release or receptor responsiveness.

Substance P

This is a small polypeptide of eleven aminoacids, which is widely distributed in the body with localisation in the central and peripheral nervous systems. Levels are highest in the hypothalamus, thalamus, basal nuclei and in the dorsal columns and roots of the spinal cord. Its role in central nervous activity is still obscure, but there is some evidence that in the spinal cord it may be involved in pain transmission while in the brain it may modulate neuronal activity and reduce pain sensitivity.

Transmitter synthesis, release, uptake and metabolism

Although very little is known of the synthesis, release and metabolism of transmitters within the central nervous system, a considerable amount of information has been obtained in recent years about the handling of acetylcholine and noradrenaline at peripheral synapses, and it is probable that similar mechanisms apply centrally. For convenience, present knowledge regarding noradrenaline in sympathetic neurones will be discussed in more detail and, where appropriate, extrapolation from this to other transmitters such as acetylcholine, dopamine and 5HT, will be made.

Noradrenaline is present in sympathetic nerve terminals in several stores or pools, being localised in terminal ramifications of the neurone which have a beaded, varicose appearance. Adrenergic neurones in the brain have a similar appearance. Approximately 40 per cent of the noradrenaline is free in the cytoplasm and the the other 60 per cent is in intra-granular stores, called 'synaptic vesicles', where it is bound to protein and hence is relatively resistant to metabolising enzymatic activity. Noradrenaline diffuses freely from the vesicles into the cytoplasm and from the cytoplasm through the cell membrane into the extracellular space. It is carried in the opposite direction by active transport mechanisms from the extracellular space to the cytoplasm, and from the cytoplasm into the vesicles. Binding of noradrenaline to protein within the vesicles probably represents a separate active process in which adenosine triphosphate (ATP) is involved.

There are two sources of the noradrenaline in the vesicles and cytoplasm:

1 Local synthesis from phenylalanine
2 Uptake from the extracellular space of noradrenaline which may either have been released locally, or have come from distant sites such as the adrenal medulla, or have been administered exogenously.

When isotopically labelled noradrenaline is injected intravenously into animals it rapidly disappears from the circulation. About half of it is metabolised, while the rest is actively taken up by adrenergic fibres and can be demonstrated radiographically in the cytoplasm and granules. When a post-ganglionic sympathetic nerve is cut and allowed to degenerate, its ability to accumulate exogenous noradrenaline disappears.

An understanding of noradrenaline uptake is important from the point of view of its inactivation after it has acted at the receptor site, for its binding within the cell represents a way in which it can be inactivated and used again.

The enzymatic metabolism of noradrenaline is largely dependent on two groups of enzymes: monoamine oxidase (MAO) and catechol-O-methyltransferase (COMT).

Monoamine oxidase is widely distributed throughout the body; within the brain it is present in larger quantities in the hypothalamus than elsewhere. It is concerned with the metabolism of a wide variety of compounds, including noradrenaline, dopamine and 5HT, and is located intracellularly in mitochondria at synaptic nerve endings, being partly responsible for regulating the cytoplasmic levels of these amines.

Catechol-O-methyltransferase is also widely distributed in brain tissue, and S-adenosylmethionine which is its cofactor is formed in the brain. Unlike MAO, it is responsible for the extracellular metabolism of noradrenaline which has diffused passively through the cell membrane or that which is released by nerve stimulation or drugs, and of catecholamines released from the adrenal medulla.

The steps in the metabolic degradation of noradrenaline, dopamine and 5HT are shown overleaf:

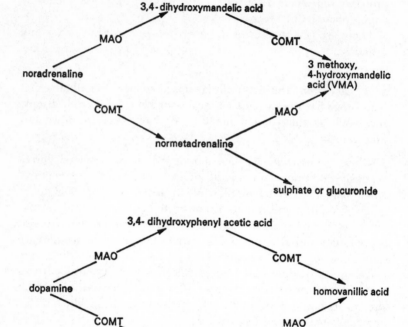

It seems likely that when a nerve impulse arrives at the end of an adrenergic neurone, storage particles of bound noradrenaline, or synaptic vesicles, fuse with the neuronal cell membrane under the influence of calcium ions which enter the cell, and then discharge their contents into the 'synaptic cleft' or extracellular space. The released noradrenaline stimulates receptors on the effector cell surface, and is then either taken up again into the pre-synaptic neurone, or is metabolised outside the cell by COMT, or is carried away by extracellular fluid.

The series of events which have been described for noradrenaline probably apply to other transmitters. 5HT is synthesised within brain neurones from its precursor tryptophan and is metabolised by MAO. It is probably stored, and released in a similar manner to noradrenaline, and there appears to be a similar uptake process for this amine. Acetylcholine is synthesised from choline within brain neurones, and is rapidly destroyed on release by acetylcholinesterase. When acetylcholinesterase is inhibited there is some evidence of an uptake process for acetylcholine also.

Presynaptic inhibition and facilitation

There is good evidence that, as well as stimulating receptors on the post-synaptic cell surface, the neurotransmitter stimulates receptors on the presynaptic membrane, and that this acts, through a negative feedback mechanism, to regulate its further release. The evidence is strongest for noradrenaline and dopamine, but may also apply to the other neurotransmitters. Blockade of these presynaptic inhibitory receptors results in facilitation of neurotransmitter release.

Receptors

Neurohumoral agents and transmitters such as those which have been described earlier in this chapter are composed, like other drugs, of molecules. The result of their action on post-synaptic cells must eventually be explained in terms of an interaction of these molecules, or parts of them, with specific molecules on the post-synaptic cell membrane. The latter are called the 'specific receptors' for the transmitter or drug with respect to the particular effect. The term 'receptor' is usually limited to drug-cell or transmitter-cell combinations that initiate a sequence of specific effects. Other drug-cell or transmitter-cell interactions that do not initiate these specific effects, such as binding of drugs to plasma, binding of neurotransmitter to cell protein and to enzymes for transport, storage and biotransformation, are referred to in other terms such as 'secondary receptors', 'storage sites', or' drug acceptors'.

Little is known of the chemistry of receptor substances in the central nervous system. It is possible to make certain tentative suggestions on their nature, however, on the basis of what is known about their counterparts in the peripheral autonomic system. Much of our knowledge of these has been gained from studies using specific receptor-blocking drugs, but often these drugs do not pass readily into the brain from the vascular system and so their usefulness in studying central receptors is limited.

Cholinergic receptors

The peripheral autonomic effects of acetylcholine are similar to those produced by the alkaloid muscarine and thus are known as its 'muscarinic actions', as distinct from its actions on ganglia and neuromuscular junctions which resemble those of nicotine, the so-called 'nicotinic' actions. Microinjection of acetylcholine into the brain and spinal cord, and studies in whole animals and isolated tissues with the tremor-producing compound oxotremorine, suggest that central cholinergic receptors are predominantly muscarinic and are blocked by compounds which block muscarinic receptors such as atropine and hyoscine. However, in several areas of the brain and spinal cord there is evidence of nicotinic receptors, or of receptors which appear to be intermediate between the nicotinic and muscarinic type.

Adrenergic receptors

In 1948, Ahlquist suggested that the effects of adrenaline at peripheral sympathetic sites could be divided into two groups with two types of receptor, alpha and beta. These were originally called 'excitatory' and 'inhibitory' receptors, respectively, because of their general tendency to produce excitation or inhibition when stimulated, but as there are important exceptions to this in both groups, it is better to refer to them only as alpha and beta receptors. Noradrenaline has predominantly alpha-adrenergic activity, the most important in man being vasoconstriction of arterioles in the skin and splanchnic area, producing a rise in systemic blood pressure, dilatation of the pupil and relaxation of the gut. The beta actions are mimicked by the synthetic sympathomimetic drug isoprenaline and include acceleration of the heart, dilatation of arterioles supplying skeletal muscles, bronchial relaxation and relaxation of the uterus. Drugs which selectively block alpha actions are known as adrenergic alpha receptor blocking drugs and include phenoxybenzamine, phentolamine, thymoxamine and tolazoline. The adrenergic beta receptor sites may be blocked selectively by a variety of related drugs including propranolol, oxprenolol, pindolol, alprenolol and sotalol. No sympathomimetic drug yet available has pure alpha or beta stimulating actions. When the alpha receptor effects of noradrenaline are blocked, for example by thymoxamine, its weaker beta receptor actions are seen, and even the potent beta receptor agonist compound, isoprenaline, can be shown to have weak alpha stimulating properties when its beta receptor actions are blocked with propranolol. Presynaptic receptors (page 21) appear to be of both alpha and beta type;

stimulation of the alpha receptors inhibits further noradrenaline release, while presynaptic beta receptor stimulation facilitates it. Presynaptic alpha receptor blockade facilitates, and beta receptor blockade inhibits, noradrenaline release.

Although the alpha and beta receptor actions appear to be so different, it is probable that the actual receptor substance is the same, namely adenylcyclase. This enzyme catalyses the conversion of ATP to cyclic AMP, and is widely distributed in a large number of animal tissues.

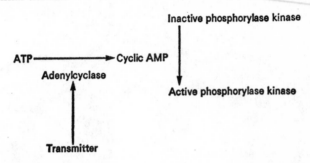

Catecholamines, such as adrenaline, noradrenaline and iso-prenaline, have a central stimulating action, which gives rise to anxiety and restlessness; this stimulating action is probably due, at least in part, to stimulation of central receptors, through the same adenylcyclase-receptor mechanism as in the periphery.

Other receptors

Relatively little is known of the nature of the receptors in the central nervous system with which 5HT, dopamine and other transmitters might react. Indeed, there is controversy as to whether each transmitter has its own specific receptors, or whether the same receptor enzyme, or different parts of it, interacts with more than one transmitter. However, there seems to be good evidence that 5HT and dopamine, at least, have their own specific receptors in the central nervous system.

In the peripheral autonomic system it appears that there are at least two types of 5HT receptor, one of which is preferentially blocked by morphine (M receptor); the other is blocked by dibenzyline (phenoxybenzamine) (D receptor). Lysergic acid diethylamide (LSD) inhibits D receptor activity, but not M receptor activity. It is too early to be certain if central 5HT receptors correspond to one or both of these types, although there is some preliminary evidence that they are more likely to be D receptors.

Dopamine has some peripheral effects, for example on the renal arteries, which suggest that there are specific dopaminergic receptors and that it does not necessarily act through stimulating noradrenaline receptors.

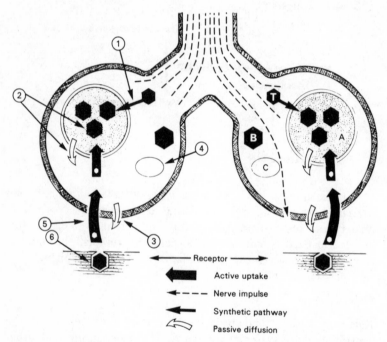

Figure 2 *Diagrammatic representation of a central monoaminergic synapse showing possible sites of drug action*
Right: A, granular pool of monoamine. B, cytoplasmic pod of monoamine. C, monoamine oxidase. T, precursor of monoamines (tyrosine, etc.)
(Modified from P. Turner and A. Richens, in *Clinical Pharmacology*, 1973, by kind permission of Churchill Livingstone.)

Mechanisms of the action of psychotropic drugs

From this brief review of the probable pharmacological basis of central nervous transmission, it is evident that a drug may interfere with central nervous function in a variety of ways (see Figure 2):

a   Inhibition of synthesis of transmitter substances
b   Production of 'false transmitter'
c   Increased precursor load
d   Depletion of transmitter from neurones
e   Inhibition of release of transmitter
f   Release of transmitter from neurones on to receptor
g   Monoamine oxidase inhibition
h   Uptake inhibition
i   Receptor stimulation
j   Receptor blockade

Inhibition of transmitter synthesis (site 1)

Several compounds are known to block the synthesis of one or more transmitters in animals, but little is known of their effects in man.

The synthesis of noradrenaline in man is inhibited by at least two substances which are used clinically. Alpha-methylparatyrosine inhibits the conversion of tyrosine to dopa by the enzyme tyrosine hydroxylase, which is the rate-limiting step in noradrenaline biosynthesis. This reduces tissue levels of noradrenaline, but 5HT levels remain unchanged. When used clinically in the management of patients with phaeochromocytoma, alpha-methylparatyrosine tends to produce sedation, while mild anxiety and insomnia often appear after sudden withdrawal of the drug.

Alpha-methyldopa is an antihypertensive agent which also reduces tissue levels of noradrenaline. This effect is due, in part, to inhibition of dopa decarboxylase, interfering with the conversion of dopa to dopamine. The enzyme is also concerned in the production of dopamine, histamine and 5HT, and levels of these transmitters in tissues such as the brain and heart are reduced at the same time as noradrenaline. Sedation occurs in almost all patients treated with methyldopa, but tends to disappear as treatment continues. When the drug is discontinued, a transient 'release-type' phenomenon of increased activity, excitability and insomnia may occur.

The biosynthesis of 5HT in the brain is inhibited by p-chlorophenylalanine which blocks tryptophan hydroxylase activity, the rate-limiting enzyme for 5HT synthesis. Its behavioural effects are not marked, and administration of large doses to experimental

animals does not appear to produce consistent stimulant or inhibiting effects. However, pre-treatment with p-chlorophenylalanine interferes with the characteristic pharmacological effects of
other drugs, such as LSD, which interact with 5HT mechanisms
in the brain. Its effects in man are not yet known.

Production of false neurotransmitter (site 1)

A drug may be taken up into a nerve cell and metabolised so that it
replaces the normal transmitter and is later released on nerve
stimulation or by other drugs. The effects of such drugs on the
receptors may either be similar to or different from those of the
physiological transmitter substances. There is evidence that alpha-
methylnoradrenaline stimulates central alpha adrenergic receptors
in the nucleus of the tractus solitarius or in the vasomotor centre,
which mediate reduction in sympathetic outflow, and so lower
blood pressure.

The antihypertensive drug alpha-methyldopa already referred
to in the previous section is thought to act in part by competing
with dopa for decarboxylation by dopa decarboxylase so that the
following biosynthesis occurs:

Alpha-methyldopa ——►Alpha-methyldopamine ——►Alpha-methylnoradrenaline

Alpha-methylnoradrenaline, therefore, replaces noradrenaline in
equimolar concentrations in adrenergic neurones and may be released by nerve impulses as a false transmitter with noradrenaline
(the physiological transmitter). Experimental evidence from animals
and man on the relative activity of noradrenaline and alpha-
methylnoradrenaline is inconsistent, but it seems unlikely that the
central and antihypertensive effects of alpha-methyldopa can all
be explained in terms of a false transmitter action of alpha-
methylnoradrenaline.

There is considerable evidence that amphetamine, after releasing noradrenaline, is metabolised in nervous tissue to p-hydroxy-
norephedrine. This compound, which may then replace noradrenaline in adrenergic neurones, has less receptor stimulant
activity than noradrenaline or alpha-methylnoradrenaline. The
formation of p-hydroxynorephedrine with its lesser stimulant
action may thus account in part for the tolerance which develops
to the central and peripheral effects of amphetamine.

After inhibition of monoamine oxidase, endogenous tyramine, which is normally metabolised by this enzyme, accumulates in neural tissue together with its hydroxylated derivative octopamine. The latter accumulates in nerve endings in the brain, as well as peripherally, and is released by nerve stimulation to act as a false transmitter in competition with noradrenaline. The extent to which any of the behavioural changes, induced by monoamine oxidase inhibition, are due to the effects of octopamine is not yet known.

Increased precursor load (site 1)

Administration to an animal or man of a precursor of a neurotransmitter substance may lead to increased synthesis of the transmitter, provided that rate-limiting steps in the synthetic pathway are not already fully loaded. Thus, administration of levodopa orally or parenterally leads to an increase of dopamine in the basal ganglia and of noradrenaline in some other tissues.

Tryptophan administered orally is hydroxylated to form 5-hydroxytryptophan which in turn is decarboxylated to 5-hydroxytryptamine.

$$\text{tryptophan} \xrightarrow[\text{hydroxylase}]{\text{tryptophan}} \text{5-hydroxytryptophan} \xrightarrow{\text{decarboxylase}} \text{5-hydroxytryptamine}$$

Similarly histidine is the precursor of histamine and is readily converted to it by the enzyme histidine decarboxylase.

Possible clinical implications of the use of some of these precursors will be described in later chapters.

Depletion of transmitter from neurones (site 2)

Reserpine is an alkaloid obtained from the roots of *Rauwolfia serpentina*, a climbing shrub indigenous to India and neighbouring countries. More than twenty alkaloids can be extracted from this plant with a wide variety of pharmacological actions, the most important of which is the depletion of tissue stores of noradrenaline, adrenaline, dopamine, 5HT and histamine, particularly in the brain. This depletion probably involves inhibited binding of these monoamines in the intracytoplasmic granular stores so that they are more vulnerable to monoamine oxidase activity. The amine-depleting action results in two important therapeutic effects, namely the calming of manic and schizophrenic patients, and an antihypertensive effect in patients with hypertension. These therapeutic actions may easily become serious unwanted effects, however, for further amine depletion can itself produce severe depression (see chapter 7). Whether this is due to specific depletion of either noradrenaline or 5HT, or of both together, is not yet certain. Its dopamine-depleting effects result in parkinsonism which may be accompanied by choreoathetosis and cerebellar ataxia.

Alpha-methyldopa is another compound which produces depletion of noradrenaline, dopamine, 5HT and histamine from the brain. At least two mechanisms for this have already been described, namely inhibition of synthesis, and replacement of the physiological transmitter by a 'false' one. This depletion probably accounts for the sedation and depression which commonly occur with its use, and for the parkinsonism which may be seen with high doses over long periods of time.

Inhibition of release of transmitter (site 3)

Some antihypertensive drugs such as bretylium, bethanidine, debrisoquine and guanethidine are thought to interfere with peripheral sympathetic nerve activity by preventing release of noradrenaline from the nerve ending. They do not have significant behavioural effects in antihypertensive doses, possibly because of their failure to penetrate the brain. It is unlikely that any psychotropic drugs now in use act predominantly by this mechanism.

Release of transmitter from neurone on to receptor (site 3)

Sympathomimetic amines, which mimic the effects of sympathetic stimulation, may be broadly divided into two groups (see Table 1).

Table 1 *Classification of sympathomimetic amines into predominant direct and indirect activity*

Directly-acting	Adrenaline
	Noradrenaline
	Dopamine
	Isoprenaline
	Phenylephrine
	Methoxamine

Table 1—*Contd.*

Indirectly-acting	Amphetamine
	Ephedrine
	Hydroxyamphetamine
	Phenmetrazine
	Tyramine

The first group of catecholamines comprising adrenaline, noradrenaline, isoprenaline and dopamine, together with some other amines such as phenylephrine, depend mainly for their effects on direct stimulation of adrenergic receptors. The second group depend mainly for their effects on their ability to be taken up into the sympathetic nerve terminal and then to release noradrenaline from the synaptic vesicles in the nerve ending on to the receptor. They are, therefore, called 'indirectly acting' sympathomimetic compounds. This distribution is easily demonstrated in the peripheral autonomic system, for example in the eye, where depletion of noradrenaline by sympathectomy or drugs such as reserpine or high concentrations of guanethidine leads to abolition of the mydriatic effects of ephedrine, tyramine, amphetamine and phenmetrazine while the effects of phenylephrine and adrenaline persist.

It is probable that the central actions of amphetamine, phenmetrazine and other indirectly acting amines also depend on the liberation of noradrenaline and dopamine from central adrenergic and dopaminergic neurones. Animal experiments have shown that the central stimulant action of dexamphetamine is almost completely blocked by pre-treatment with reserpine, and by compounds which inhibit noradrenaline and dopamine synthesis. Its activity is restored, however, by very small doses of dopa which have no effects in the normal animal. The relative importance of dopamine and noradrenaline in mediating various components of the central effects of amphetamine is still not certain. The problem is complicated by the possible 'false transmitter' role of metabolites of amphetamine such as p-hydroxynorephedrine, already described.

It may well be that other centrally acting drugs act in part or whole by releasing one or more transmitter substances from central neurones.

Monoamine oxidase inhibition (site 4)

Inhibition of the action of the intracellular enzyme monoamine oxidase (MAO) leads to an accumulation within the nerve of monoamines such as noradrenaline, dopamine, 5HT and histamine. This occurs both peripherally and centrally. Monoamine oxidase is in fact a general term for a series of more specific enzymes which deal with the individual monoamines, but MAO inhibitors tend to inhibit the whole family of enzymes, and thus lead to an increase in all the amines. A large number of drugs inhibit MAO to a limited extent, including cocaine and amphetamine, but their main actions do not appear to depend on this property. In the case of other compounds, including the hydrazine derivatives iproniazid and phenelzine and the amphetamine derivative tranylcypromine, their pharmacological actions probably do depend on MAO inhibition. The hydrazine group produce a long-lasting inhibition by an irreversible, non-competitive inhibition of the enzyme *in vitro* and *in vivo*. In contrast, the harmala alkaloids, harmine and harmaline, produce a short-lasting, reversible competitive inhibition of the enzyme.

Inhibition of MAO enhances the elevation of brain catecholamine and 5HT concentrations and the central stimulation produced by precursors of these transmitters. It also reverses the central depression and amine-depleting effects of reserpine, and enhances the central stimulant effects of drugs such as amphetamine which release central stores of noradrenaline.

Uptake inhibition (site 5)

Uptake of noradrenaline into the adrenergic nerve terminals represents a major route of its inactivation, and it is probable that a similar mechanism operates with other transmitter substances including dopamine and 5HT. Inhibition of this uptake would lead to an increase in the activity of transmitter at the receptor site.

A large number of drugs have been shown to interfere with noradrenaline uptake, including many with actions on the central nervous system. Among these are the central stimulant compounds amphetamine and cocaine, the antidepressant drugs imipramine and tranylcypromine, and the tranquillising drugs chlorpromazine and reserpine. Because of the wide spectrum of clinical effects shown by drugs which possess this action it is probable that, in the case of most of these compounds, inhibition of uptake, though an interesting pharmacological phenomenon, does not contribute to the primary clinical effect. In the case of the dibenzazepine drugs, however, such as imipramine, it is probable that inhibition of uptake with increase of transmitter at the receptor site plays an important role in its main therapeutic action. Furthermore, it has been suggested that at least part of the central action of the phenothiazine compounds, such as chlorpromazine, is the result of partial blockage of noradrenaline uptake at sites where the latter is acting as an inhibitory transmitter, so leading to a potentiation of its inhibiting effects.

It might be argued that facilitation of uptake with increase of intraneuronal breakdown of noradrenaline by MAO could lead to a decrease in the concentration of transmitter at central receptor sites. This, in fact, is one of the suggested modes of action for lithium salts in the prophylaxis of manic depressive psychosis (see chapter 7).

While inhibition or facilitation of monoamine uptake into animal brain slices can be readily demonstrated, studies in man are largely limited to the use of changes in noradrenaline or tyramine pressor effects as a measure of noradrenaline reuptake, and to changes in platelet dopamine and 5-HT uptake. It appears that, under certain carefully controlled conditions, the human platelet may be a useful model for screening the effects of drugs on the uptake of these two amines into central neurones.

Receptor stimulation (site 6)

Some compounds may exert their central effects by a direct stimulation of central receptors. Apomorphine, bromocriptine and piribedil are thought to stimulate dopamine receptors, and the tremor-producing compound, oxotremorine may stimulate central cholinergic receptors.

Receptor blockade (site 6)

Many drugs are known to block specifically adrenergic, cholinergic and 5HT receptors in the peripheral autonomic system, and it is probable that the central actions of some compounds are due to a similar mechanism. For example, the sedating effects of hyoscine may well be due to central cholinergic receptor blockade. It is probable also that phenothiazine drugs, such as chlorpromazine, owe the major part of their central effects to a dopamine receptor-blocking action, and the same may be true of the butyrophenones such as haloperidol. It is tempting to apply similar reasoning to the antihistamine compounds by suggesting that their central effects are due to histamine-receptor blockade in the brain.

It is evident that there are several different ways in which a compound may produce central nervous effects when considered in terms of its interactions with neuronal processes at the trans-mitter level. Many compounds may have several different actions. For example, chlorpromazine has been shown in different experimental procedures to influence the release of noradrenaline, to affect its uptake into the neurone, and to block dopaminergic receptors. It is difficult to be certain which, if any, is the most significant. Similarly, the MAO inhibitors have a marked effect on the uptake, as well as the breakdown, of noradrenaline, and it is uncertain on which of these two actions their central stimulant effects depend.

Another example is that of propranolol, the beta adrenoceptor blocking drug which in low plasma concentrations of about 100 ng/ml acts predominantly by blocking beta receptors, but in higher concentrations of 1000 ng/ml and above, which are reached with the doses used in antipsychotic studies, probably has local anaesthetic, membrane stabilising and 5 HT inhibiting actions. Furthermore, the foregoing discussions has centred around the acute effects of drugs on the synthesis, release and uptake of transmitter substances and on receptor activity. Other factors, however, may be important:

1 *Regional variations in the site of action* For example, pheno-thiazines are thought to act primarily in the brain stem region, and benzodiazepines in the limbic system, while barbiturates probably act in a more diffuse and non-specific manner through the cortex and subcortical structures.

2 *Presynaptic inhibition and facilitation* See page 21.

3 *Longer-term changes in monoamine activity* Feedback mechanisms on the rate of transmitter synthesis and in receptor activity are known to occur in response to the acute changes produced by drugs which have been described. In particular, receptor blockade tends to be followed by increased transmitter synthesis and release,

and uptake blockade by reduced synthesis and release. It has also been shown that long-term changes occur in the intracellular concentrations of cyclic AMP in response to changes in synaptic levels of neurotransmitter, and these may have important implications in terms of clinical responses to drugs.

4 *Membrane and intracellular processes* (other than those already discussed) Compounds may interfere with neuronal cell membrane activity and ion transport, so reducing the ability of the transmitter substance to trigger-off impulses in the post-synaptic cell. Other drugs may interfere with energy-releasing enzyme systems, so producing their effects beyond the receptor. Drugs which interfere with transmitter mechanisms may also affect these other, less well defined factors, and so their actual mode of action is even more difficult to define.

Suggestions for further reading

BRADLEY, P. N., 'The pharmacology of synapses in the central nervous system', in *Recent Advances in Pharmacology*, ed. J. M. Robson and R. S. Stacey, Churchill, London, 1968.

COSTA, E., and GARATTINI, S., *International Symposium on Amphetamine and Related Compounds*, Raven Press, New York, 1970.

CUELLO, A. C., POLAK, J. M., and PEARSE, A. G. E., 'Substance P: a naturally occurring transmitter in human spinal cord', *Lancet*, vol. 2, 1976, p. 1054.

D'AVIES, D. A., and REID, J. L., *Central Action of Drugs in Blood Pressure Regulation*, Pitman Medical, Tunbridge Wells, 1976.

HORNYKIEWICZ, O., 'Parkinson's disease and its chemotherapy', *Biochemical Pharmacology*, vol. 24, 1975, pp. 1061–5.

IVERSEN, L. L., *The Uptake and Storage of Noradrenaline in Sympathetic Nerves*, Cambridge University Press, 1967.

IVERSEN, L. L., IVERSEN, S. D., and SNYDER, S. H., *Biogenic Amine Receptors* (Handbook of Psychopharmacology, vol. 6), Plenum Press, New York, 1975.

JOHNSON, A. M., LOEW, D. M., and VIGOURET, J. M., 'Stimulant properties of bromocriptine on central dopamine receptors in comparison to apomorphine, (+) amphetamine and l-dopa', *British Journal of Pharmacology*, vol. 56, 1976, pp. 59–68.

LANCET (Editorial), 'Substance P', *Lancet*, vol. 2, 1976, p. 1067.

PHILLIS, J. W., *The Pharmacology of Synapses*, Pergamon Press, Oxford, 1970.

SNYDER, S. H., 'Neurotransmitter and drug receptors in the brain', *Biochemical Pharmacology*, vol. 24, 1975, pp. 1371–4.

VETULANI, J., and SULSER, F., 'Action of various antidepressant treatments reduces reactivity of noradrenergic cyclic AMP—generating system in limbic forebrain', *Nature*, vol. 257, 1975, pp. 495–6.

Factors influencing the action of psychotropic drugs

3

It is a fact of clinical experience that there is considerable variation from patient to patient in the response to a fixed dose of almost any drug. Such variation is at least partly due to the fact that the blood level of a drug following a given dose can vary by more than tenfold from one patient to another. It is not surprising, therefore, that in any patient population a given dose of a drug may produce a satisfactory therapeutic response in some, absence of effect in others, and evidence of intoxication in a further group. A number of factors are responsible for this phenomenon, apart from the obvious one of failure to take the prescribed dose of the drug (see chapter 5). The rate of absorption of the drug, its distribution throughout the body, its binding to plasma proteins and to tissues, its rate and routes of metabolism and excretion, all influence its concentration at the site of action and hence its clinical effects. Pharmacokinetics is the name given to study of these aspects of pharmacology, and rational prescribing depends on an understanding of pharmacokinetic principles.

Drug absorption

Following oral administration, a drug has to cross the bowel wall somewhere along its length to enter the circulation. Substances cross the gut mucosa in one or more of the following ways:

1 passive diffusion, which depends upon the concentration gradient
2 active transport against a concentration gradient by an energy-consuming mechanism
3 filtration through pores
4 pinocytosis, by which small particles are engulfed by mucosal cells.

The first mechanism, passive diffusion, is the most important for drug absorption, and is influenced by several different factors:

A *The chemical nature of the drug* Most commonly-used drugs are either weak acids (e.g. aspirin, barbiturates) or weak bases (e.g. amphetamine, tricyclic antidepressant drugs of the mono-amine reuptake inhibitor type), (MARI), and these exist in two forms in solution, namely, as undissociated molecules and as ions. The equilibrium between these two forms is determined by (i) the pH of the surrounding medium, and (ii) the pK value of the drug. At a pH equal to the pKa the drug is 50 per cent ionised. At a low pH, for example in the stomach, a weakly acidic drug is mainly in its undissociated form whereas a weakly basic drug will be largely ionised. The reverse applies in an alkaline medium such as occurs in the small bowel.

In general, the undissociated molecules are more lipid soluble than the ionised species, and are thus more readily absorbed across the complex lipid membrane which is the gut mucosa. An alkaline medium, therefore, favours absorption of the weakly basic drugs.

B *Formulation* When a drug is prescribed the patient actually receives a medicine. The active substance may represent only a small proportion of the total weight of an oral solid dosage form such as a tablet or capsule. In recent years it has become increasingly realised that the other constituents of dosage forms are not necessarily inert but may facilitate or hinder a drug's absorption. Among the important factors involved in the production of tablets and capsules which may influence a drug's absorption are:

(i) Particle size of the drug. It was a change in particle size that produced the marked change in bioavailability of digoxin in Britain in the early 1970s.

(ii) Diluents, such as lactose or calcium sulphate which are used to increase bulk. A change in diluent led to an outbreak of phenytoin intoxication in Australia.

(iii) Granulating and binding agents, such as tragacanth, syrup or bentonite which assist aggregation of the powder into granules in order to permit compression into tablets.

(iv) Lubricants, such as talc, prevent granule adherence to the tableting machines.

(v) Disintegrating agents such as starch and cocoa butter are incorporated to produce rapid tablet disintegration in the gastro-intestinal tract.

(vi) Coating materials such as sugar or the gelatin envelopes of capsules may prevent breakdown before the preparation reaches the stomach.

(vii) Special formulations employ complex pharmaceutical processes to control the rates of disintegration and dissolution and so to regulate the rate of a drug's absorption, for example in sustained-release formulations.

C *Gastric emptying and gut motility* Most drugs are absorbed from the upper part of the small bowel, and drugs which delay gastric emptying, particularly those with anticholinergic activity such as amitriptyline or imipramine, can delay their own absorption and that of other drugs. Metoclopramide, which increases the rate of gastric emptying, may produce more rapid absorption of another drug given at the same time.

D *Bowel wall and liver enzymes* Unless a drug is absorbed directly into the systemic circulation, as from sublingual or rectal administration, it has to pass through the liver in the portal circulation. Furthermore, the gut mucosa also possesses some drug metabolising activity. Thus, when the indirectly acting sympatho-mimetic amines ephedrine or tyramine are ingested orally they are normally metabolised by the enzyme monoamine oxidase in the gut wall and liver. This enzyme is inhibited by monoamine oxidase inhibitors, allowing the passage of these substances into the systemic circulation (see page 42). Hepatic enzyme induction, on the other hand, can lead to increased metabolism of drugs in their passages through the liver (see pages 42 and 155).

Distribution and protein binding

The lipid solubility of a drug not only influences its rate of absorption across the gut mucosa, but also its distribution throughout the body. A strongly basic drug such as the ganglion blocking drug hexamethonium is poorly absorbed from the gut, and when given parenterally, remains largely in the extracellular fluid. The blood-brain barrier consists of the vascular wall of the cerebral circulation and the tissue in contact with it. This is predominantly a lipid membrane which behaves very much like the gut wall as far as passive diffusion is concerned. Therefore, drugs which are well absorbed from the gut are usually able easily to enter the brain. This presupposes, of course, that the drug is not completely metabolised as it passes through the liver into one or more compounds which are less lipid soluble and so less able to cross into the brain. A high degree of lipid solubility is a characteristic of centrally-acting drugs, including anaesthetic agents both volatile, and non-volatile such as thiopentone. These drugs, however, for the same reason, can easily cross the placenta to the foetal circulation, and it was a centrally acting drug (thalidomide) which produced such tragic teratogenic effects.

Most drugs are bound, to a greater or less degree, to plasma and tissue proteins. The extent of binding is important, as it is generally only the unbound drug which is biologically active. Therefore, in the case of a highly-bound drug, the biological activity resides in only a small proportion of the total plasma level, and a relatively small increase in the unbound fraction may produce a marked increase in therapeutic or toxic activity. Such an increase may result from:

1 a change in concentration of plasma proteins, particularly albumin (in hypoproteinaemic states a higher level of unbound drug occurs in the plasma unless the oral dose is lowered)
2 displacement of bound drug from binding sites on proteins by other drugs.

Metabolism

Most drugs are metabolised to some extent in the liver, although, in addition, some are destroyed by enzymes in the plasma and other tissues. Liver metabolism occurs particularly with lipid soluble drugs, which may be taken up so avidly by the liver that a total extraction occurs from the blood during its first passage through the portal circulation after absorption.

The best known example of this 'first pass' phenomenon is propranolol in which between 20 and 40 mg of an oral dose is removed by the liver. Until this hepatic extraction is saturated, little, if any, parent drug is able to reach the systemic circulation. Other drugs with important first-pass effects include morphine and lignocaine.

The object of drug metabolising activity is to produce derivatives of increasing polarity which are less lipid soluble and so more readily excreted by the kidney. Drugs possessing a hydroxyl, carboxyl or amino group are usually conjugated to form a glucuronide, an ethereal sulphate, or a glycine or acetyl derivative. Drugs lacking one of these groups are usually oxidised, dealkylated, deaminated or hydroxylated, and subsequent conjugation often occurs. It is important to remember that a metabolite of a drug may be pharmacologically and therefore therapeutically active, and that its profile of activity may differ from that of the parent drug. This is demonstrated in the case of the tertiary amines amitriptyline and imipramine which are demethylated to the secondary amines nortriptyline and desipramine respectively, both of which are antidepressant drugs, but differ in their pharmacological properties from the parent compounds.

Differences in rates of drug metabolism account for most of the differences in steady-state blood level already referred to. For example, steady-state levels of some MARI antidepressant drugs vary up to 20 or 30 fold on a fixed daily dose, most of this variability being due to differences in rates of hydroxylation, while inter-patient differences in protein binding and tissue distribution are two-fold or less.

Acetylation depends on the activity of the enzyme N-acetyl transferase, the concentration of which is genetically determined. The population can be divided into fast and slow acetylators, and this has been shown to influence the therapeutic and toxic effects of a variety of drugs including isoniazid and procainamide. It has recently been shown that the monoamine oxidase inhibitor phenelzine undergoes acetylation and that clinical response to this drug may depend upon the acetylator status of the patient.

Excretion

Most drugs, or their metabolites, are excreted in the urine, and the same principles apply to passive diffusion through the renal tubule as were discussed earlier with regard to drug absorption. The ionised species of a drug is less lipid soluble and so does not readily diffuse back from the glomerular filtrate through the renal tubular wall into the circulation. Therefore, changes in tubular pH can influence the rate of elimination of weakly acidic or basic drugs and their metabolites. Normally the urine is slightly acid and favours the excretion of weakly basic drugs such as amphetamine, pethidine and tricyclic antidepressants. The reverse applies for weakly acidic drugs, and this is the reason why an alkaline diuresis is used to accelerate the elimination of aspirin and some barbiturates (see chapter 16).

Because the kidney is the main organ of excretion for many drugs, care must be exercised in prescribing drugs for patients with impaired renal function.

Some drugs are excreted mainly in the bile, and may then be reabsorbed from the small bowel to produce an 'entero-hepatic' circulation. Drugs and their metabolites, particularly glucuronide conjugates, are liable to biliary excretion if they are polar and if their molecular weights exceed 400.

Blood levels

Following the absorption of a drug from the gut or from a site of parenteral administration, and its distribution to the tissues, its concentration in the plasma or serum falls along an exponential time course. A semi-logarithmic plot of concentration versus time produces a straight line relationship from which can be obtained the half-life ($t\frac{1}{2}$) of the drug, that is, the time taken for the concentration to fall to half of its original level. The half-life, when absorption and distribution is complete, is determined by those processes of metabolism and excretion already described.

The concept of half-life is a valuable one in deciding the frequency of drug dosage. Levodopa, for example, has a short half-life and requires at least four divided doses daily to produce a steady plasma level and therapeutic action. On the other hand, amitriptyline has a half-life of 30–40 hours, and only requires a once-daily administration. The development of a special 'sustained-release' form of this drug for once-nightly administration was, therefore, quite unnecessary. Drugs with a long half-life may be cumulative with repeated and frequent dosage, and patients receiving them should be examined carefully and regularly for signs of overdosage.

The foregoing considerations with respect to blood levels of a drug and its elimination half-life are only of clinical importance when there is a close and temporal relationship between plasma concentration and pharmacological or therapeutic effect. In the case of some centrally acting drugs this clearly applies, for example with lithium. With many others there appears to be a relationship, but it is not so clear-cut, for example with phenothiazine neuro-leptics and antidepressant drugs of the monoamine reuptake inhibitor type (MARI). This may be because being very lipid soluble, they reach high concentrations in different parts of the brain, which do not necessarily correlate closely with plasma levels in concentration or time. Finally, there are other drugs whose mechanism of action renders it unlikely that such a close relationship could be found, for example, the monoamine oxidase inhibitors.

Other factors

Several other factors are recognised which influence drug action, either by effects on the pharmacokinetic variables already mentioned, or by effects on tissue response.

Age has a marked influence on metabolism and excretion particularly at the extremes of life in infancy and old age. Old age brings a reduction in liver metabolising activity and in renal excreting ability. It is also associated with changes in distribution of body tissues, for example, the proportion of body fat. Changes in the cerebral circulation associated with increasing age may also contribute to differences in response to centrally acting drugs seen in elderly patients.

Sex differences almost certainly influence drug activity. Female patients show considerable differences in pressor response to sympathomimetic amines at different times of the menstrual cycle, and this may also apply to central monoamine receptors. Sex differences have been observed in the central stimulation produced by anorectic drugs, which may be due to pharmacokinetic factors as well as to differences in receptor activity.

Drug interactions involving psychotropic drugs

Patients receiving drug treatment for a psychiatric condition are usually receiving more than one drug at the same time, and these may interact in a variety of ways for the patients; either for good or for harm. The following is a summary of some of the mechanisms by which such interactions may take place.

1 *Absorption*

Drugs which influence the rate of gastric emptying may modify the rate of absorption of other drugs. Anticholinergic activity, in particular, slows the rate of gastric emptying, and this property is shared by several groups of psychotropic drugs including the MARI antidepressant drugs, the phenothiazines, and the anticholinergic antiparkinsonian drugs. Their effect is to delay passage of the drugs into the small bowel, and thus, most commonly, to delay their systemic absorption.

Gut wall and liver monoamine oxidase normally destroys mono-amines such as tyramine which is present in food (e.g. in cheese and other foods subject to microbial action) as well as sym-pathomimetic substances such as phenylephrine which are sub-strates for the enzyme and are found in proprietary and other medicines used as nasal decongestants and in coryza. Treatment with monoamine oxidase inhibitors reduces the activity of this enzyme and so permits the systemic absorption of such mono-amines, with the risk of a hypertensive reaction.

2 *Hepatic enzyme induction*

The magnitude and duration of action of many drugs, as well as endogenously produced substances, are dependent on their rate of biotransformation by the drug-metabolising enzymes of the liver. The activity of these enzymes may be increased, or induced by treatment with a large number of commonly used substances including insecticides and pesticides, and also by drugs, chiefly the barbiturates, glutethimide, methaqualone, phenytoin and rifam-picin. The steady-state plasma concentration of some MARI antidepressant drugs can be markedly reduced by addition of a barbiturate hypnotic to the treatment regimen. Benzodiazepines in therapeutic doses do not induce these enzymes. The state of hepatic drug metabolising activity can be assessed indirectly *in vivo* by measurement of antipyrine elimination half-lives, serum gamma-glutamyl-transpeptidase, and urinary excretion of glucaric acid and 6-β-hydroxycortisol.

3 *Hepatic enzyme inhibition*

The effect of monoamine oxidase inhibitors in the gut and liver has already been discussed. Clinically important inhibition of drug metabolising enzymes in the liver may occur with phenothiazines and butyrophenones which may result in reduced metabolism of MARI antidepressants, leading to higher plasma levels and enhanced effects.

4 Blockade of neuronal uptake

The active reuptake of noradrenaline into the neurone is an important mechanism in its termination of action. Blockade of the reuptake process potentiates the pressor action of noradrenaline and adrenaline, and of other drugs that depend on the same uptake process, such as phenylephrine. This may be important in administration of local anaesthetic preparations containing one of these amines as a vasoconstrictor. Among the groups of drugs which may block neuronal uptake are the MARI antidepressants such as amitriptyline and imipramine, and their metabolites nortriptyline and desipramine. Some indirectly acting sympathomimetic amines, such as tyramine, and some adrenergic neurone blocking drugs such as guanethidine, bethanidine and debrisoquine, depend for their pharmacological and therapeutic effects on being taken up into the neurone through the same active uptake process as noradrenaline. Their action may, therefore, be prevented or reversed by treatment with MARI antidepressant drugs. Phenothiazines also possess uptake-blocking properties and may have similar effects on these antihypertensive drugs.

5 Transmitter depletion

The effects of drugs which depend for their action on release of certain transmitter substances may be reduced by administration of other drugs which produce neurotransmitter depletion. For example, pressor responses to tyramine are reduced in reserpinised patients.

6 Functional summation of effects

Drugs which produce a similar pharmacological effect by different mechanisms may have a synergistic interaction, for example the mutual enhancement in the central nervous system of the depressant activity of hypnotics, sedatives, tranquillisers, alcohol, narcotic analgesics and anaesthetics.

There may also be summation of the same pharmacological effect of several drugs given for different purposes. For example, phenothiazine neuroleptics, many MARI antidepressants, and antiparkinsonian drugs such as orphenadrine and benzhoxol all possess anticholinergic properties which may summate if a member of each group is given together for acceptable psychiatric

43

and neurological indications, to produce a central anticholinergic crisis.

This crisis with its psychological concomitants is sometimes mistaken for worsening of the psychiatric condition for which the psychotropic drugs are being administered; if this happens then higher doses may be prescribed, with potentially disastrous results.

Table 2   *Clinically important interactions involving psychotropic drugs*

Primary drug A	May interact with B	Potential results
Monoamine reuptake inhibitor antidepressant (MARI)	Bethanidine Debrisoquine Guanethidine Clonidine	Reduction of antihypertensive action of B
	Monoamine oxidase inhibitors	Central nervous excitation, hyperpyrexia, coma
	Anticholinergics Antihistamines Antiparkinsonian drugs	Excessive central and peripheral atropine-like effects
	Noradrenaline Adrenaline Phenylephrine	Potentiation of pressor action of B
	Any orally-administered drug	Change in absorption of B
	Phenothiazines and butyrophenones	Potentiation of hypotensive effect of B
Monoamine oxidase inhibitors (MAOI)	Indirectly-acting sympathomimetics Fenfluramine Levodopa Foods containing tyramine	Acute adrenergic hypertensive crisis
	MARI anti-depressants	Central nervous excitation, hyperpyrexia, coma

Table 2—*Contd.*

Primary drug A	May interact with B	Potential results
	Pethidine	Central nervous excitation, coma
Anxiolytics		
Benzodiazepines	Alcohol Other CNS depressants	Increased CNS depression
Barbiturates	Coumarin anticoagulants	Reduced activity of B.
	Corticosteroids	Reduced effect of B in asthma
	Oral contraceptives	Contraceptive failure
	Other CNS depressants	Increased CNS depression
	MARI anti-depressants	Reduced plasma levels and ? effect
Beta-adrenoceptor blocking drugs	Antihypertensive drugs	Increased hypotensive action
	Insulin Sulphonylureas	Increased hypoglycaemic action of B
	Skeletal muscle relaxants (depolarising)	Increased activity of B
Hypnotics	Alcohol Narcotic analgesics Antihistamines MARI anti-depressants Phenothiazines Butyrophenones	Increased CNS depression

Table 2—*Contd.*

Primary drug A	May interact with B	Potential results
Phenothiazines and butyrophenones	Alcohol Narcotic analgesics Other CNS depressants	Increased CNS depression
	Anticholinergics MARI anti-depressants	Impaired oral absorption of A Enhancement of peripheral and central anti-cholinergic effects
	MARI anti-depressants	? enhanced effect of B through hepatic enzyme inhibition
	Bethanidine Debrisoquine Guanethidine	Reduction of antihypertensive action of B
Lithium	Diuretics	Lithium retention and toxicity
	Sodium chloride	With reduced sodium intake, lithium retention. With increased sodium intake, greater lithium excretion

Suggestions for further reading

Pharmacokinetics

CURRY, S. H., *Drug Disposition and Pharmacokinetics*, Blackwell, Oxford, 2nd edn, 1977.

DAVIES, D. S., and PRICHARD, B. N. C., *Biological Effect of Drugs in Relation to their Plasma Concentration*, Macmillan, London, 1973.

LADER, M., 'Clinical psychopharmacology' in *Recent Advances in Psychiatry*, ed. K. Granville-Grossman, Churchill Livingstone, Edinburgh, 1975, pp. 1–30.

JOHNSTONE, E., and MARSH, W., 'Acetylator status and response to phenelzine in depressed patients', *Lancet*, vol. 1, 1973, p. 567.

SCHANKER, L. S., 'Physiological transport of drugs', in *Advances in Drug Research*, ed. N. J. Harper and A. B. Simmonds, Academic Press, London, 1965, vol. 1, p. 71.

SMITH, S. E., and RAWLINS, M. D., *Variability in Human Drug Response*, Butterworths, London, 1973.

TURNER, P., and RICHENS, A., *Clinical Pharmacology*, 2nd edn, Churchill Livingstone, Edinburgh, 1975.

WAGNER, J. G., *Fundamentals of Clinical Pharmacokinetics*, Drug Intelligence Publications, Hamilton, Illinois, 1975.

VESSELL, E. S., 'Pharmacogenetics', *Biochemical Pharmacology*, vol. 24, 1975, p. 445.

Drug interactions

GRIFFIN, J. P., and D'ARCY, P. F., *A Manual of Adverse Drug Interactions*, Wright, Bristol, 1965.

LAURENCE, D. R., 'Important interactions of antidepressive drugs', in *Advanced Medicine—Topics in Therapeutics*, ed. P. Turner, Pitman Medical, Tunbridge Wells, 1975, vol. 2.

SMITH, S. E., and RAWLINS, M. D., *Variability in Human Drug Response*, Butterworths, London, 1973.

TURNER, P., and RICHENS, A., *Clinical Pharmacology*, 2nd edn, Churchill Livingstone, Edinburgh, 1975.

WADE, O. L., and BEELEY, L., *Adverse Reaction to Drugs*, 2nd edn, Heinemann, London, 1976.

4 Methods of studying behavioural effects of drugs

In most other areas of clinical pharmacology the therapeutic effects of a new drug may be predicted with some confidence on the basis of animal experiments alone. However, in psychopharmacology it is difficult to predict behavioural effects in man from findings obtained in animals. This is because:

1 there are few, if any, satisfactory animal models of abnormal human mental states such as schizophrenia, depression, mania or anxiety.

2 it is often impossible to be certain whether objective changes in animal behaviour after administration of a drug are due to sensory or motor effects, or both, or to changes in co-ordination, or even to hallucinatory effects.

In fact, it may not be possible to detect any therapeutic drug effect at all until the compound is given to patients suffering with a particular condition. For example, levodopa has few, if any, central effects in normal subjects but can readily be seen to affect motor activity in patients with Parkinson's disease. Similarly, the anti-depressant activity of the MAO inhibitors and dibenzazepine compounds can only be detected in patients with established depression. Although valuable clues may come from various animal tests, these tests often appear to bear little relation to clinical conditions in man.

In this chapter, tests will be briefly described which may be used to detect and evaluate central actions of drugs in animals and man, particularly those drugs to which reference will be made in later sections of the book.

Animal tests

There are a very large number of animal tests used to screen the effects of drugs on the central nervous system, and to study their mechanism of action. They can be classified in three main groups:

1 Pharmacological and biochemical
2 Behavioural
3 Electroneurophysiological

1 *Pharmacological and biochemical tests*

These include biochemical and histochemical studies of animal brain tissue to demonstrate localisation of possible transmitter substances and the influence of drugs upon them, as well as test procedures involving isotopically labelled drugs, such as auto-radiography (to show the distribution of a drug within various organs) and tracer studies (to determine the metabolic pathway of a drug).

A commonly used test for screening potential antidepressant compounds makes use of reserpine-induced hypothermia. Administration of reserpine to an animal reduces its body temperature, probably by monoamine depletion. MAO inhibitors and dibenzazepine derivatives, known to have antidepressant activity in man, reverse this hypothermic effect of reserpine. On the other hand, some other types of antidepressant drugs such as mianserin do not possess this property.

2 *Behavioural tests*

There are a large number of tests in which the effects of drugs on animal behaviour may be observed. Many involve operant or classical conditioning procedures and may require a complex experimental design. One of the simplest behavioural tests is the Y maze in which an animal has to make a choice between the two limbs of the Y; the action of drugs on this choice can be measured and added effects of reward or punishment observed.

A rather more dramatic procedure is that measuring the 'muricidal activity' of cats, in which a mouse is released into a cage with a cat and the behaviour of the latter is observed.

Analgesic tests, of which there are a formidable number, may be considered to be behavioural, as it is now generally accepted that 'pain' represents a response of the whole organism to a noxious stimulus (see chapter 14).

3 Electroneurophysiological tests

Neuronal activity within the brain and spinal cord is accompanied by changes in electrical potential across the cell membrane. The summation of these changes in large numbers of neurones may be recorded by superficial electrodes placed on the scalp, as in electroencephalography, a technique widely used in human studies. In animals it is possible to implant electrodes in specific areas of the brain, or even localise them to individual cells, and so record electrical events more discretely.

A sophisticated modification of this principle involves introducing a minute amount of pharmacologically active substance in the vicinity of a neurone through a micropipette controlled by micromanipulators, and recording the potential changes produced with adjacent microelectrodes. Multichannel micropipettes have been developed by drawing out a number of glass tubes fixed together. The multichannel micropipette made in this way has closely adjacent openings at the common tip, the central channel of which may be used as a recording electrode, while the secondary pipettes can be used for the introduction of substances whose actions are to be tested. For recording extracellular potentials in the brain it is preferable to use electrodes with a tip diameter of 6μ or less.

As well as recording electrical changes in the brain and spinal cord, implanted electrodes may be used to stimulate discrete areas and study the effects of such stimulation on the animal's behaviour and physiology. The influence of drugs on such responses to electrical stimulation may then be investigated.

Tests in man

Sensory tests

1 *Smell and taste* Smell thresholds may be determined by delivering into the nose, through rubber or plastic catheters, metered doses of a test substance such as coffee or xylol. The number of doses necessary to produce a recognised sensation of smell of the test substance is taken to be the threshold dose. Taste thresholds may be measured by presenting a series of substances in ascending concentrations to the tongue, the subject being asked to report what he tastes. These tests lack the sensitivity of tests of some other modalities, but when carried out under carefully controlled conditions, can reveal consistent changes in olfactory acuity

brought about by central-stimulant compounds such as amphetamine and phenmetrazine.

2 *Vision* A test of visual function which is mediated by the central nervous system, and is most useful in the monitoring of drug effects on the brain, is the critical flicker frequency (CFF). This may be defined as the fastest rate at which a flashing source of light appears to be flickering as opposed to being steady. It has a number of determinants including the luminance, wave-length, wave-form and light–dark ratio of the stimulating light; the area, portion and light-adapted state of the retina illuminated; the duration of exposure, and the size of the pupil. Age and constitutional factors may also influence the threshold and recently the importance of intersensory effects has been recognised.

By rigorously controlling these many variables in the experimental situation it has been possible to use the test for assessing the effects of central depressant and stimulant drugs. Alcohol produces a marked depression of CFF which is porportional to the alcohol concentration in blood and urine. Barbiturate drugs depress CFF and dose response effects may be obtained starting with doses as low as 50 mg amylobarbitone. Anxiolytic sedatives, such as meprobamate, chlordiazepoxide and diazepam, as well as phenothiazine drugs, lower CFF in doses which are too small to produce any subjective awareness of central depression.

Central stimulant drugs such as amphetamine and phenmetrazine increase CFF, as do hallucinogenic stimulant compounds such as psylocybin. Combinations of barbiturates and amphetamines in appropriate proportions may show mutual antagonism of effects on CFF. Thus, a mixture of dexamphetamine and amylobarbitone in the proportions found in Drinamyl produces no change in CFF when compared with placebo, although dexamphetamine alone produces a rise and amylobarbitone a fall in threshold. Measurement of CFF over a period of time allows a study of the duration of action of drugs and the influence of physiological variables on it. For example, the rate of excretion of amphetamine is markedly dependent on urinary pH, a low pH resulting in rapid elimination of the drug and an alkaline urine delaying its excretion. A comparison of the duration of action of amphetamine on CFF under conditions of urinary acidity and alkalinity showed that the magnitude and duration of elevation of CFF was significantly greater under alkaline than under acid conditions.

51

Drugs may also affect the peripheral components of vision such as extraocular motor balance, pupil and lens function and rod and cone activity involved in colour vision.

3   *Hearing*   Just as the critical flicker frequency is a measure of a subject's ability to distinguish an intermittent light source, so the auditory flutter-fusion threshold (AFFT) is a measure of central auditory function. An interrupted random noise signal is used, and although the threshold varies greatly from subject to subject, it is very constant for any one person if measured, like the CFF, under strictly controlled conditions. Amylobarbitone 100 mg, diazepam 10 mg and chlorpromazine 25 mg and 50 mg significantly depress the AFFT, while amphetamine 10 mg raises it.

4   *Pain*   There are a large variety of tests designed to measure pain thresholds in normal man, most of which are unsatisfactory and fail to show changes after administration of analgesic drugs in clinically effective doses.

Thermal stimuli have been applied, using hot and cold objects, but this method has many inherent variables such as the pressure of the warm or cold object and absorption of the heat by blood flow through the skin, which may itself be altered by the thermal stimulus. The use of radiant heat is also subject to this variation of local skin blood flow.

Electrical stimulation of the skin and tooth pulp has been widely used; it may discriminate between therapeutic doses of analgesics, such as aspirin and morphine, and identical placebos. There are large variations in threshold within subjects, however, and the skin and the pulp method may produce a hyper-irritable state which can persist for months. It is also possible to block dental pulp pain non-specifically, for example by adrenaline, which may confuse tests of centrally acting drugs.

The most predictable and sensitive methods of producing experimental pain involve causing muscle ischaemia with a tourniquet to occlude arterial flow in a limb, followed by exercise of that limb. The pain produced by this technique can be so intense that subjects may be very reluctant to repeat the tests on other occasions unless motivation is very high.

The intraperitoneal instillation of bradykinin to produce pain has been used in human volunteers, and has permitted determination of dose-response curves with non-narcotic and narcotic analgesic drugs, but its potential dangers are such that the method cannot be recommended for routine screening.

We should distinguish between pain threshold and pain tolerance. The former relates to the detection of a painful stimulus, the latter to the length of time for which this can be borne. Placing the hand in a water bath kept at a constant temperature of 10°C is in itself not particularly unpleasant to begin with, but it soon becomes quite painful. It is relatively simple to measure the time the subject can keep his hand in such a water bath; this determines pain tolerance. Drugs can affect threshold and tolerance differently.

Measurement of pain in disease is different from measurement of experimental pain. Pathological pain carries with it the implications of a potent threat to the patient's physical integrity; the nature of the stimulus is often unknown and the severity of the pain is modified by the patient's psychological characteristics.

Several methods are used for measuring pathological pain:

(a)   Simple descriptive pain scale in which points are allocated to pain of different intensity, for example 0–4 may represent the range: no pain, slight, moderate, severe and agonising pain.

(b)   Matching methods, in which patients attempt to match the severity of their pathological pain against an experimentally-induced pain, such as thermal stimulus.

(c)   Non-verbal methods such as squeezing a bag or moving a lever in proportion to the severity of the pain.

(d)   Visual analogue scale (see page 58).

. Of these various methods, the visual analogue scale seems to be the most sensitive, both for measuring pain and assessing response to treatment.

Tests of co-ordination and motor function

It is difficult to draw fine distinctions between sensory, motor and co-ordination tests in man, for even the sensory tests already described require a response from the subject which involves some co-ordination and motor activity. Nevertheless, in the tests previously described, the emphasis was mainly on sensory activity, whereas in the tests described in this section, attention is focused primarily on motor skills and on co-ordination of motor with sensory activity. It may not be easy to distinguish, however, between effects of drugs on local neuromuscular and spinal activity, and effects on the brain.

1   *Reaction time*   This is the time taken for a subject to record a response to a given stimulus. In an alert subject this time may be very short, and electronic timing devices may be required to give a sufficiently accurate measurement. Even before the introduction of such equipment, however, it was possible to obtain results which showed effects of central depressant drugs. Almost a century ago Lauder Brunton used a system of pendulums and levers to demonstrate the effects of alcohol and other drugs on central function. It is customary to present the subject with a number of stimuli, both visual and auditory, in random order, and instruct him to respond to one particular stimulus by depression of a morse key or other form of electrical switch.

2   *Disc dotting*   In this test of co-ordination, in which the McDougal–Schuster machine is most commonly used, a subject cancels, with a pencil, an irregular spiral of dots within circles as it rotates slowly on a turntable. Vision is restricted by covering the spiral with a lid in which there is only a small radial aperture. The cancellations begin at the origin of the spiral at the centre of the turntable and continue until the subject misses two consecutive target circles; the score comprises the number of 'dots' in the track up to the point where it has been broken.

A modification of this method consists of a rotating metal drum covered with an insulating layer in which holes have been cut in an irregular spiral course. The subject uses a steering-wheel to follow the course of holes with a lever and thus establishes electrical contact with them; the score is recorded on a digital counter. Drugs such as promethazine when given in single doses, have been shown to reduce performance significantly.

3   *Ball bearings*   In this test of manual dexterity, the subject is required to pick up ball bearings (3 mm diameter) from a dish, using a pair of fine curved forceps, and then to drop the ball bearings, one at a time, into a small vertical glass tube with an internal diameter of about 4 mm. The score is the number successfully transferred to the tube in a given time.

4   *Tapping speed*   This is a test of both co-ordination and motor ability, in which the subject taps on a morse key as rapidly as possible for a given period of time; a counter registers the number of contacts made.

5 *Hand steadiness*   There are a variety of test situations designed to measure hand steadiness. Most require the subject to hold a metal rod or ring in close proximity to another metal object, such as a plate or wire, or to move one along the other, without allowing the two to touch. Contact of the metal objects completes an electrical circuit which can activate a bell, buzzer or light. The apparatus may be designed to give the subject a harmless but unpleasant shock when this happens.

6 *Pursuit rotor*   In this test a point light source moves rapidly on a screen and the subject attempts to follow it with a rod at the end of which is a photoelectric cell. This records the amount of time for which the subject is able to keep the rod in contact with the light source and hence the accuracy of this movement.

7 *Reverse mirror drawing*   This is a measure, not only of a subject's co-ordination, but also his sense of lateralisation. He sees the image of a design, such as a star, in a mirror in front of him, but the design itself is hidden by a screen. He is required to follow the outline of the design with a pencil held below the screen, controlling it from the mirror image. The time taken to complete the test, and the number of errors made, are recorded.

Psychological rating scales

Psychotropic drugs are usually prescribed for the relief of emotional distress or the amelioration of a disturbed mental state; two conditions which are very difficult to measure directly. To determine the relative efficacy of such drugs in these clinical situations we have to rely on a variety of rating scales, and other psychometric tests, a number of which are available. They fall into four broad categories:

1 Tests of intelligence and other cognitive functions
2 Scales designed to quantify overt behaviour
3 Ratings based on a standardised clinical interview
4 Self-rating scales completed by the patient himself

1 *Intelligence tests and other tests of cognitive function*   These are perhaps the most familiar of all psychological measuring devices having been in use for over fifty years. Essentially, they attempt to

55

quantify the ability of the subject to solve standardised problems and to learn new information. They are particularly useful in cases of suspected organic disease of the brain, and the most commonly used are the Wechsler Adult Intelligence Scale (WAIS), the progressive matrices, and the Mill Hill Vocabulary Test.

2 *Overt behaviour scales* These scales are among the earliest introduced for specifically psychiatric purposes. Among the first was the Phipps Psychiatric Clinic Behaviour Chart introduced in 1915 for nurses to use in making a daily numerical assessment of a variety of behaviours exhibited by their patients on the ward. A more recent example of this type of scale is in the Nurses' Observation For In-patient Evaluation (NOSIE).

The disadvantages of such measures are: first, they can be used only on hospital in-patients, and then only in a ward where the numbers and training of the nursing staff are adequate; and second, they afford very little information on subjective phenomena such as emotions, perceptions and beliefs.

3 *Clinical rating scales* These are basically designed to provide a quantitative estimate of the findings obtained during a clinical interview. There are two types, each having a somewhat different aim:

(i) Scales designed to provide information over a wide range of possible symptoms; they are useful as an aid to diagnosis
(ii) Scales which are primarily intended for estimating changes in individual symptoms occurring in specific psychiatric disorders.

While the second group of scales is only valid after a diagnosis has been made, it does allow more critical evaluation of drug changes within the particular given diagnostic grouping under study.

The complexity of rating scales of the first type ranges from the sixteen-item *Brief Psychiatric Rating Scale* to the '*Present Psychiatric State' Examination* covering over 400 items.

Of the scales designed to assess change occurring as a result of treatment within specific diagnostic groups, the most widely used include:

(i) *The Hamilton Anxiety Scale* in which twelve symptoms commonly associated with the diagnosis of anxiety state plus an

impression of behaviour at interview are rated on a five-point scale
(0=absent, 1=mild, 2=moderate, 3=severe, 4=very severe,
5=grossly disabling).

(ii) *The Wing Scale for Schizophrenia* in which four attributes of
schizophrenia, flatness and incongruity of affect, poverty of speech,
incoherence of speech and coherent delusions are each rated on a
four-point scale.

(iii) *The Hamilton Depression Scale* in which twenty-four features
of depressive illness are separately considered and rated.

A variant of the specific diagnostic type of scale is the overall
rating in which the clinical condition under study is rated as
absent, mild, moderately severe, severe, extremely severe. In the
global evaluation of drug treatment this is often as good as any of
the more detailed scales considered above.

4 *Self-rating scales* With this type of scale, which does not
require the presence of either a doctor, a psychologist or a nurse,
the patient himself completes it by answering a series of multiple-
choice questions. Here is a sample question from a self-rating scale
used in the assessment of depression, the *Beck Depression Scale*
(only one of the following statements must be marked as reflecting
the patient's feelings):

0   I do not feel sad.

1. I feel blue and sad.

2a I am blue and sad all the time and I can't snap out of it.

2b I am so sad or unhappy that it is very painful.

3   I am so sad or unhappy that I can't stand it.

Another widely used self-rating scale for depression is the *Zung
Scale*.

A number of self-rating scales for anxiety exist; the most widely
used are the *Taylor Manifest Anxiety Scale* (TMA) and the
Institute of Personality and Ability Testing (IPAT); however, a
more recently developed scale, the *Morbid Anxiety Inventory*
(MAI), appears to be more sensitive for measuring drug effects.

While such scales are obviously open to evasion or exaggeration
by patients, in practice they are extremely useful and are economi-
cal of professional time.

The major difficulty encountered by patients completing such scales is the inability to decide upon one particular answer or category. (These scales are often referred to as *category scales*.) This is especially true of the Yes/No-type scales such as the *Eysenck Personality Inventory* (EPI) a very widely used measure intended to obtain an assessment of personality in terms of neuroticism, extraversion and introversion.

A recent innovation which avoids this difficulty is the *Analogue Scale* consisting of a straight line, usually 100 mm long, with one end labelled, for example, 'not at all anxious' and the other 'extremely anxious'. The labels can vary according to the condition or sensation being evaluated. Patients are asked to mark the line at the point which most appropriately reflects their state at the time. While there is considerable variation in the way different people use such a scale, it allows a very sensitive assessment of change occurring within a given person, and is particularly useful in monitoring drug effects.

Choice of rating scale

The choice of rating scale for any given project depends partly on the purpose for which it is to be used, and partly on the clinical condition to be studied. It is in most cases a compromise between exhaustiveness and exhaustion. If a great deal of information is required about a relatively small number of patients, and there are sufficient trained personnel to administer the scale, then the Present State Examination is without doubt the most comprehensive available instrument. However, most clinical studies of psychotropic drugs require relatively large numbers of patients and take place in clinics and hospitals where staff time is at a premium. Therefore for out-patient and general practice investigations the self-rating scales are probably the most useful. Their value is obviously much less in conditions such as severe depressive illness or schizophrenia where patient co-operation cannot be relied upon. It is particularly among these populations, usually in an in-patient setting, where the standardised clinical rating scales, like the Hamilton Anxiety and Depression Scales, and the Wing Scale for Schizophrenia apply.

Finally, it should be stressed that there is no intrinsic numerical value in the scores obtained by any of these scales; they merely enable a clinical impression or a subjective feeling state to be quantified. They do not actually measure anything directly.

Psychophysiological tests

Many psychiatric disorders are accompanied by physical mani-festations. Centrally acting drugs may affect these manifestations, or may themselves have direct effects on various physiological activities. Only a brief review of some of the test procedures used in this field of psychophysiological measurement will be attempted here.

1 *Heart rate and blood pressure* Heart rate and blood pressure may be abnormal in psychotic conditions, such as depression, mania and anxiety. Centrally acting drugs may also produce changes in these parameters, either through their central effect or through other peripheral actions which they possess.

In some circumstances it may be sufficient to record pulse rate by simply counting the radial pulse for a minute, and to measure blood pressure by the standard sphygmomanometer technique, after the subject has rested for at least five minutes. However, for a more accurate assessment of drugs on central and peripheral autonomic function, it is preferable to use electrical recording devices. While a standard electrocardiogram (ECG) will provide sufficient data to record heart rate, it does not provide the informa-tion in a useful way. By employing electronic circuits to perform the operations involved in heart beat recognition, counting and timing, by using a cardiotachometer, the need to count individual ECG complexes is avoided.

Automated recording of systolic and diastolic levels of blood pressure is more difficult, and in fact, there are few, if any, accurate methods which do not depend on arterial catheterisation, although systolic blood pressure alone may be recorded with rather simpler techniques. A commonly used method involves occlusion of the blood supply to a finger, using a small cuff. The point of occlusion is then determined by testing for a pulse distal to the cuff by means of: (i) a second cuff connected to a sensitive volume-displacement transducer, (ii) a small finger plethysmograph, (iii) a small crystal transducer strapped to the finger tip, (iv) by observing changes in optical density of the finger tip photoelectrically. Refinements of these methods permit continuous and automatic recording of systolic pressure.

2 *Skin conductance and skin potential* When a small electric current is passed between two points on the surface of the skin the conductance varies with the state of the subject's mental state. Measurements of the skin conductance levels are usually made over the palm; they often show slow and gradual changes as a function of the changing mental state of the individual; in the case of sleeping or drugged subjects the conductance may rise markedly, while the conductance falls rapidly following specific arousing stimuli.

Measurement of skin conductance changes are of considerable value in psychopharmacology, including the so-called psychogalvanic response (PGR) in which there is a change in conductance occurring as a result of a psychological stimulus. The technique is not simple, however, for the voltage and conductance involved is small, and requires sophisticated electronic recording apparatus and intimate electrode-skin contact to obtain accurate measurement. In addition, the stimuli used must be carefully controlled in order to keep arousal levels as constant as possible. Furthermore, it should be remembered that changes in skin conductance can occur with drugs which influence sweat gland function by a purely peripheral action.

3 *Plethysmography* Plethysmography consists of enclosing an organ in a rigid container called an oncometer and measuring the volume changes of the enclosed part. This permits study of the nervous and chemical control of blood flow into the organ and changes in that blood flow induced by disease or drugs.

There are many different kinds of plethysmograph, but those used in psychopharmacology usually involve recording pulsatile variations in the volume of a finger or the forearm. Although these measurements of variations in organ volume are not direct estimations of rate of blood flow, under certain strictly controlled conditions, which usually involve sudden occlusion of the venous drainage, the pulse volume is a close index of the rate of blood flow.

Plethysmography is used particularly in studies of anxiety, mania and depression, in which physiological changes in blood flow can be demonstrated, and in the effects of drugs in these conditions.

Penile plethysmography is a variant of the method in which volume changes of the penis during erection can be determined by measuring the changes in a mercury-filled loop placed around the penis. This technique is of particular value when assessing the effect of various treatments on sexual responsiveness, as, for example, in the treatment of sexual deviance by cyproterone (see chapter 12).

4 *Electromyography* Tension of a muscle at rest can be a valuable indicator of the mental state of a subject, particularly in conditions of stress and agitation. Although direct measurement of muscle tension in man is difficult, the electrical changes which accompany muscle activity can be recorded; it is also possible to record muscle tremor by suitable modification of the procedure. Electromyograms are usually obtained from surface electrodes placed over appropriate muscle groups but may be complicated by artefacts which make interpretation difficult. An alternative method is to use needle electrodes, but the major difficulty here is that only a very small volume of muscle tissue is sampled by the electrode tip and its precise localisation may not be easy to determine.

5 *Electroencephalography* A detailed discussion of the changes which can occur in the electroencephalogram (EEG) in mental and neurological disease, or in response to drugs, is beyond the scope of this book. Many physiological and metabolic variables influence the EEG and considerable experience is required to recognise changes which are due to extraneous factors. However, the EEG changes produced by certain groups of drugs are so consistent that their presence in a record can be considered as a strong indication that such drugs have been taken. Stopping drugs, particularly when the subject has become habituated to them, may also affect the EEG in important ways. For example, paroxysmal discharges may be seen in a significant proportion of subjects following barbiturate withdrawal, even in the absence of any previous history of epilepsy.

Because of the large number of variables which may modify the EEG, the following strictly controlled conditions are required for recording:

1 Complete routine EEG assessment, including sleep records, should be made on all supposedly normal subjects before admission to a study
2 All records should be taken by the same recordist

3 The same EEG apparatus should be used throughout
4 Subjects should be investigated at the same time of day and at the same time interval after the previous meal
5 Females should be investigated at the same stage of the menstrual cycle
6 Recording techniques should be standardised
7 Quantitative measurements based on short samples of the EEG should be made at a constant time interval after eye closure or eye opening.

It is most convenient to use electronic methods of frequency analysis and summation to demonstrate changes in the EEG. A valuable additional technique measures 'evoked potentials', which are EEG responses evoked by specific stimuli such as visual or auditory signals. Many evoked potentials are of low amplitude and obscured by spontaneous background activity. However, as they are of a constant pattern, frequency analysis and summation procedures allow them to be picked out more clearly. The influence of drugs on these evoked potentials is of considerable interest.

6 *Pupillometry* Changes in pupil size are continuously taking place in association with alterations in mood and response to emotional stimuli. Arousal and fear produce pupillary dilatation while revulsion and disgust produce contraction. Centrally acting drugs, as well as drugs which modify peripheral autonomic activity, may also influence pupil size.

The pupil is supplied by both sympathetic and parasympathetic divisions of the autonomic nervous system and its diameter is readily measurable by photographic and other methods. Its responses to drugs, such as cholinergic and sympathomimetic substances, are consistent in repeated determination within subjects under standard conditions.

There are several methods available for measuring pupil responses. When rapid changes in diameter are being recorded, and when pupillary reactivity to light and dark are also being observed, infra-red pupillography is the most convenient. Infra-red light is reflected from the retina through the pupil, and is then monitored continuously on a recording apparatus, to show pupillary contraction and dilatation.

Where slower responses are being studied, however, this is often unnecessary and simpler photographic methods are equally acceptable; photographs of the eyes are taken and pupil diameter measured from the negatives after suitable magnification.

Among the centrally acting drugs which have been studied in this way, dibenzazepine derivatives such as imipramine produce pupil dilatation due, in part, if not completely, to reduced parasympathetic activity. Phenothiazines, butyrophenones and reserpine contract the pupil to varying extents. Pupillary response to locally instilled sympathomimetic amines may be influenced by centrally acting drugs, and this may provide valuable information on their basic pharmacological actions. For example, oral reserpine treatment reduces or may even abolish the mydriatic action of the indirectly acting amine ephedrine, amphetamine and tyramine while leaving the direct effects of phenylephrine unchanged. On the other hand, treatment with monoamine oxidase inhibitors potentiates the mydriatic actions of the indirectly acting amines.

7 *Feeding behaviour* Feeding behaviour and appetite are affected in many psychiatric conditions and influenced by a number of centrally acting drugs (see chapter 13). Hunger can be reliably assessed with a visual analogue scale (see above). Food intake, on the other hand, while easier to measure directly, presents technical difficulties of application. Many studies on food intake have in fact been limited to the measurement of liquid nutriments such as Metercal (Metrecal). Recently, however, a food dispenser has been developed which allows of the continuous monitoring of the intake of solid foods presented in acceptable standard aliquots.

Clinical trials

In psychiatric disease states, where there are virtually no appropriate animal models, potential therapeutic compounds can only be fully evaluated in patients. In addition, as there are so relatively few parameters in these conditions which can be measured accurately enough to assess the effects of drugs, and as the natural history may be unpredictable, it becomes difficult to relate change in clinical state to the effects of the treatment given.

For all these reasons it is important to design well-controlled clinical trials in order to evaluate the action of centrally acting drugs in psychiatry.

Clinical trials may broadly be divided into two types, the pilot trial and the controlled trial.

1 *Pilot clinical trial* In this type of trial, which may include the first administration of a new drug to man, a relatively small number of subjects are studied in depth. The drug is first administered in very small doses to normal subjects, or to patients, with informed consent having been obtained either from the subject or from responsible relatives. Test procedures such as those already described in this chapter are carried out before and at intervals after administration of the drug, together with toxicological studies, including haematology, liver and renal function, and electrocardiography. The toxicological tests are done at suitable times to show acute effects and to reveal any delayed hypersensitivity reactions which may occur. Metabolic and biochemical studies provide information on the absorption, excretion and biotransformation of the drug. Careful patient observation should permit a determination of the dose necessary to produce a desired clinical effect, if such an effect be present, together with the dose which produces undesirable effects; this allows the therapeutic ratio of the drug to be determined. At the same time possible mechanisms of action are explored.

The main object of this type of trial is to obtain some experience of the new compound, particularly with regard to its spectrum of activity and its toxic effects. This is done in an 'open' way, with both the investigator and experimental subject or patient aware of the nature of the investigation and the treatment used.

Having completed this part of the study, if the investigator feels that the evidence is suggestive of a useful therapeutic effect, the following two questions should be asked before proceeding further:

(i) Has the compound significant therapeutic effects when compared with an identical placebo preparation ? (ii) Is the new treatment as good as, or superior to, the best treatment at present available ? The answer to the first question will tell whether the drug is therapeutically active when investigator and subject bias have been exluded. Even if it were active, it would have little place in clinical practice if it were shown to be inferior to treatment already available. The controlled clinical trial is an experimental technique by which reliable answers to both these questions can be obtained.

2 *Controlled clinical trial* Bias on the part of the investigator or patient is a major source of error in the assessment of psychopharmacological agents. Many studies have shown that the greater

the degree of control introduced into a trial of a new drug, and the smaller the opportunity for bias, the less enthusiastic are the claims made for it; these findings are illustrated in Table 3.

Table 3 *Effect of research design on the outcome of clinical trials**

Research design	Studies reporting less than 70% patients improving no. %	Studies reporting 70% or more improving no. %
No control groups or blind techniques	93 (42)	127 (58)
Control groups but no blind techniques	57 (54)	48 (46)
Control groups and blind techniques	66 (67)	32 (33)

* From *Psychopharmacology Bulletin*, March 1969

The most important measures taken to eliminate bias are (1) the double-blind technique (2) randomisation of treatments and (3) matching of patients.

1 *Double-blind technique* The purpose of this technique is to ensure that neither investigator nor patient is aware of the treatment which the patient is receiving. For each treatment the new drug, a standard drug and an inactive placebo, are prepared in such a way that they appear identical. This may simply mean making tablets of the same colour, shape and size, but it may also involve flavouring to match the taste, and even introducing other substances to produce unrelated drug effects. For example, if a trial of a new dibenzazepine derivative is to be really double-blind, all the treatments used should produce some impairment of accommodation, dryness of mouth and interference with micturition and bowel function.

An important consideration when preparing a double-blind trial is to ensure that the formulation of the standard drug, which is usually a compound in current use, provides the same 'biological availability' as the generally used preparation. Otherwise, another error might be introduced, loading the result unfairly in favour of, or against, the new drug. 'Biological availability' refers to the ease with which the drug can be absorbed from the gastrointestinal tract; it can be influenced markedly by the excipient substances present in the tablet or capsule to provide bulk, even though they may lack significant pharmacological activity themselves, and may not appear to influence the cruder tests of tablet disintegration and dissolution (see page 36).

2 *Randomisation of treatments* Having disguised the various treatments used in a study, it is important that the order of allocation be randomised.

Trials may be divided broadly into those (i) *within-subjects* and those (ii) *between-subjects*. In within-subject trials, all the patients receive each of the treatments being tested, and their responses to each treatment are compared to their responses to the other treatments. In between-subject investigations, each patient receives only one of the treatments under trial, and the mean responses of each group of patients receiving a particular treatment are compared to the mean responses of the other groups. Which type of trial is used depends primarily on the nature of the condition being treated. In a chronic condition, such as hypertension or rheumatoid arthritis, a within-patient study is suitable because patients may be expected to return to a similar base-line of disability when treatment is discontinued. However, in conditions which are self-limiting or cyclic in nature, such as the common cold, anxiety states or depression, this assumption cannot be made, and it is not reasonable to compare treatments within the same patient.

Randomisation of treatments is necessary in both within- and between-subjects types of trial. There are two important reasons for this:

(i) It avoids observer bias. If the investigator knows the order of administration of treatment, or that C regularly follows B which follows A, then the trial cannot be considered double-blind, even though the formulations used have been matched for factors such as colour, size and shape. Claims based on trials in which treatments with active drug and placebo were allocated alternately, have not been substantiated when trials with true randomisation were undertaken.

(ii) It minimises 'carry-over' effects. The administration of one drug may influence the action of subsequent treatments in a variety of ways and so disguise their true effects. This is particularly important, of course, in within-subject trials. It is overcome by using the 'latin square' type of randomisation. This is best explained by imagining that we have our three preparations, standard, new and placebo. Subjects are arranged in blocks of three, each of whom will have a first, second and third treatment. The latin square is so arranged that each preparation occurs once, and once only, as first, second or third treatment in any three patients, as shown:

A	B	C
B	C	A
C	A	B

It is evident that in the case of three treatments in three subjects more than one latin square is possible. For example the following is an alternative:

A	C	B
C	B	A
B	A	C

As the number of treatments and subjects increases, so the possible order of treatments increases, and the actual latin square used in any one study is decided by randomisation techniques which are best employed with the help of a statistician.

3 *Matching of patients* Among the factors that influence a patient's response to drugs are age, sex, duration and severity of the condition which is being treated. In order to obtain a valid comparison of the activities of various preparations, therefore, it is desirable to match patients within treatment groups for these various factors. This may prove impossible, however, particularly if the condition is relatively uncommon. As many factors as possible should be matched, and the limitations imposed by others which are unmatched should be recognised.

Under this heading may be mentioned variations in drug response due to differences in patients' weight. In animal experiments it is usual to give the dose of a drug on the basis of body weight, but in therapeutic practice in man this is seldom done except where toxicity is high, and dose-related. In fixed-dose studies blood and tissue levels of a drug tend to be higher in lighter subjects, and this may obviously produce differences in therapeutic response and toxicity. It may be wise, therefore, either to match patients for weight as well as the other factors mentioned, or to relate the dose to the patient's weight. In practice, however, these precautions are seldom taken, and this may account in part for the wide variations in response which are often reported in trials of centrally acting drugs. One way of monitoring such variations would be to determine the blood levels of the preparations used.

Statistical analyses

The final stage of a clinical trial is the statistical analysis of the data obtained. In the past many drugs have been introduced into clinical practice on the basis of unqualified clinical judgment on the part of a few investigators who had used the compounds in an open, un-controlled way. The purpose of the measures already discussed was to eliminate observer and patient bias as far as possible, and the mathematical handling of the results obtained is the climax of this process. Table 4 shows the difference in enthusiasm for new drugs when statistical methods were used rather than conclusions based on the global judgments of patients or doctors.

Table 4   *Effect of statistical analysis on the outcome of clinical trials**

Basis of conclusions	Studies reporting less than 70% of patients improving		Studies reporting 70% or more of patients improving	
	no.	%	no.	%
Global judgment	175	(48)	191	(52)
Statistical tests	27	(59)	19	(41)

* From *Psychopharmacology Bulletin*, March 1969

Statistical methods require numerical values which can be ana-lysed, and this is a major problem with psychotherapeutic agents. Whereas drugs such as diuretics and antihypertensive agents produce changes which can be quantified in terms of urine volume or blood pressure, anxiety and changes of mood cannot be evaluated in this way. The rating scales already described may go part of the way to resolving the problem, but they cannot be said to be entirely satisfactory, as the units used bear no constant mathematical relationship to one another. Nevertheless, where it is possible to obtain numerical values, as, for example, the number of subjects showing improvement, deterioration, or relapse, using an overall assessment, or in specific items on rating scales, then statistical techniques should be used. It is not the purpose of this book to describe them in detail, and readers are referred to specialist books on the subject, some of which are mentioned at the end of the chapter. Although simple tests such as Chi squared, Student's t and ranking methods may be sufficient where large and obvious differences between treatments are seen, more sophisticated methods are available which may show significant differences which are not so readily apparent. Particularly valuable are the multivariate techniques of analysis of variance, covariance and dispersion, which minimise differences in results due to other factors such as between-subject and between-time variations, so that the between-treatment differences may be more readily seen. Such methods of analysis are very complicated, however, particularly when several symptoms and signs are being assessed, and computer facilities are almost always essential for their use.

Where the results of treatment can only be assessed in terms of global judgment, as for example, whether a patient has improved or not improved, and where there are important ethical or other reasons for discontinuing the trial as soon as a statistically significant result is obtained, the *sequential trial* may be appropriate. This involves making preferences for one form of treatment against another, either within patients or between matched patients, and plotting these on a graph prepared from tables, once the statistical requirements for significance have been decided. When a line of significance is crossed, either for one drug against another, or for no difference between treatments, then the trial can be discontinued. For studies of centrally acting drugs, as for most types of clinical trial, a figure of 5 per cent is usually taken as being significant, so that the chances of obtaining a positive result when in fact it does not exist are less than 5 per cent; equally, the chances of not obtaining a positive result when one really exists are also less than 5 per cent.

Statistical techniques are complex, and wrong conclusions may be reached if an inappropriate one is chosen for a particular problem. For this reason, it is wise to include a statistician in the research team when preparing, prosecuting and analysing the results of a clinical trial.

Suggestions for further reading

AITKEN, R. C. B., and ZEALLEY, A. K., 'Measurement of moods', *British Journal of Hospital Medicine*, vol. 4, 1970, pp. 215–24.

ARMITAGE, P., *Sequential Medical Trials*, Blackwell, Oxford, 1960.

ARMITAGE, P., *Statistical Methods in Medicinal Research*, Blackwell, Oxford, 1971.

HAMILTON, M., *Lectures on the Methodology of Clinical Research*, 2nd edn, Churchill Livingstone, Edinburgh, 1974.

HARRIS, E. L., and FITZGEARALD, J. D., *The Principle and Practice of Clinical Trials*, Livingstone, Edinburgh, 1970.

HUSKISSON, E. C., 'Measurement of pain', *Lancet*, vol. 2, 1974, pp. 1127–30.

IVERSEN, S. D., and IVERSEN, L. L., *Behavioural Pharmacology*, Oxford University Press, New York, 1975.

LADER, M., *The Psychophysiology of Mental Illness*, Routledge & Kegan Paul, London, 1975.

MCNAIR, D. M., 'Anti-anxiety drugs and human performance', *Archives of General Psychiatry*, vol. 29, 1973, pp. 611–17.

MAXWELL, A. E., *Basic Statistics in Behavioural Research*, Penguin Books, Harmondsworth 1970.

MAXWELL, C., *Clinical Research for All*, Cambridge Medical Publications, 1973.

NICHOLSON, A. N., 'Performance and impaired performance', *British Journal of Clinical Pharmacology*, vol. 3, 1976, pp. 521–2.

ROBSON, C., *Experiment, Design and Statistics in Psychiatry*, Penguin Books, Harmondsworth 1973.

SALZMAN, C., KOCHANSKEY, G. E., and SHADER, R. I., 'Rating scales for geriatric psychopharmacology—a review', *Psychopharmacology Bulletin*, vol. 8, 1972, pp. 3–50.

SIEGEL, S., *Non-parametric Statistics for the Behavioural Sciences*, McGraw-Hill, Tokyo, 1956.

SILVERSTONE, T., and FINCHAM, J., 'Experimental techniques for the measurement of hunger and food intake in man, for use in the evaluation of anorectic drugs', in *Central Mechanisms of Anorectic Drugs* ed. S. Garattini and R. Samanin, Raven Press, New York, 1978.

SMART, J. V., *Elements of Medical Statistics*, Staples Press, London, 1971.

SMITH, J. M., and MISIAK, H., 'Critical flicker frequency (CFF) and psychotropic drugs in normal human subjects—a review', *Psychopharmacology*, vol. 47, 1976, pp. 175–82.

Social and psychological aspects of drug treatment

5

We educate our patients and their friends to believe that every or almost every symptom and disease can be benefited by a drug, some ignorant practitioners believe this.

Cabot, 1906

National patterns of psychotropic drug prescribing and attitudes

Although written over seventy years ago, Cabot's caustic observation still has considerable force today; particularly in the case of emotional distress where the number and variety of pharmacological preparations prescribed for the relief of tension and anxiety has increased at a remarkable rate in recent years. For example, in the UK during the period 1961 to 1973 the number of prescriptions issued by general practitioners for drugs classified by the Department of Health and Social Security as 'tranquillisers' more than trebled, rising from 6·2 million in 1961 to 19·1 million in 1973—see Figure 3. Yet in the same period the total number of prescriptions issued for all drugs rose only by 29 per cent, from 205 million to 264 million. A similar situation obtains in the USA. It has been estimated that almost 10 per cent of the population in both countries currently take some form of psychotropic medication each day; these drugs accounting for 15–20 per cent of all prescriptions. The cost to the community for such prescriptions is staggering, exceeding £25 million in the UK and $700 million in the USA.

The greatest proportion of such prescriptions is for anxiolytic sedative drugs of the benzodiazepine type: these account for over 70 per cent of the prescriptions for tranquillisers in the UK, constituting about 90 per cent of all anti-anxiety drugs. The pattern is similar in the USA.

71

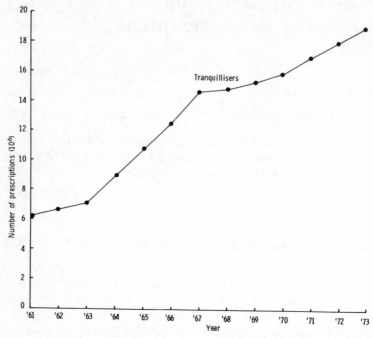

Figure 3 *Number of prescriptions issued by general practitioners for 'tranquillisers' in England and Wales, 1961–73* (from *Annual Reports, Department of Health and Social Security*, HMSO, London)

Although there has been a general increase in prescriptions for psychotropic drugs throughout the world there are considerable national and even regional variations, not only in the number of prescriptions issued but also in the attitudes to such drugs held by doctors and by potential patients. Comparable surveys of anti-anxiety/sedative drug taking have now been undertaken in ten countries under the auspices of the Psychopharmacology Research Branch of the US National Institute of Mental Health.

As can be seen in Table 5 the proportion of the population who had taken an anxiolytic sedative drug in the previous twelve months ranged from 9·7 per cent in Spain to 16·8 per cent in Belgium. The figures for the UK and the USA were 14·2 per cent and 15 per cent respectively.

In all ten countries the number of women prescribed such drugs greatly exceeded the number of men; prescribing was also more common for patients aged over 45 than for younger ones. When we look at the proportion of the population who had taken anxiolytic sedatives on a regular basis during the year the rank order is rather different; the UK comes out top, with well over 8 per cent using these drugs for a month or more, whereas it was ranked sixth among those using anxiolytic sedative drugs at all. Thus there is not only a variation in the number of patients who are prescribed these drugs, the pattern of use also varies from country to country.

Table 5 *Percentage of the adult population who had taken anxiolytic sedative drugs in the previous twelve months*

	Belgium	Denmark	France	Germany	Italy
Percentage who had used such drugs at any time	16·8	15·1	16·7	14·2	11·2
Rank order	1	4	2	6	9
Percentage who had used such drugs for one month or more	7·9	8·4	6·8	6·0	3·4
Rank order	4	2	5	6	10

	Nether-lands	Spain	Sweden	UK	USA
Percentage who had used such drugs at any time	12·7	9·7	15·8	14·2	15·0
Rank order	8	10	3	6	5
Percentage who had used such drugs for one month or more	8·1	4·0	5·0	8·6	6·0
Rank order	3	9	8	1	6

From *New England Journal of Medicine*, vol. 290, 1974, pp. 769–74.

Somewhat surprisingly the national attitudes to anxiolytic sedative drugs did not correspond particularly closely to the prescribing pattern; for example, Belgians were among the most antagonistic towards these drugs, yet Belgian doctors prescribed them more frequently than their colleagues in other countries; the Swedes were among the most favourably disposed but ranked low among regular users. In general, patients or potential patients tended to be more conservative in their attitudes towards the value of these compounds than their doctors. The majority of those questioned believed that intra-personal factors such as will-power and determination were more important than drugs in overcoming life's problems. This question is discussed further as it applies to rational drug therapy for anxiety—see chapter 8.

Drug defaulting

If an effective drug is prescribed in the informed opinion that it will ameliorate distressing symptoms, it is obviously equally important that the patient fully understands the directions for taking it and takes it as directed for as long as is considered necessary. While this may seem a naive truism, surveys have shown that many patients, particularly the elderly, have little idea of either the frequency or the number of tablets they should take, or for how long they should go on taking them. Often the prescribing doctor is unaware of his patient's failure to comply with his instructions; this can lead to accumulation of large quantities of potentially dangerous drugs in the households of such patients. An instance of this undesirable state of affairs was provided from a survey of 500 households in a town in the North of England. A total of 43,000 unwanted tablets and capsules were discovered, over a third of which were psychotropic drugs. Extrapolating from this finding to the UK as a whole it was estimated that some 1,250 million unwanted tablets or capsules are likely to be lying in cupboards and medicine cabinets. Apart from the enormous financial waste (well over £6 million) such caches of drugs are obviously a great source of danger to unwary children as well as providing a ready supply to those intent on taking an overdose.

One easily remediable cause for non-compliance among patients who are prescribed drugs by their doctor is inadequate instructions being given to the patient. It has even been said: 'In our society better instructions are provided when purchasing a new camera or automobile than when the patient receives a lifesaving antibiotic or cardiac drug.' Full and detailed instructions are particularly necessary for those of limited intelligence or whose mental powers are failing. This is especially so when more than one drug is prescribed. Visual aids may be of considerable help in imparting the relevant information and the assistance of relatives should be enlisted where possible.

Another reason for patients failing to take their drugs as intended is the development of side-effects. There is therefore little point in prescribing large quantities of tablets if the patient is going to stop taking them as soon as an undesirable side-effect develops. This is particularly true in the area of psychotropic drugs, the great majority of which can produce such effects.

A further cause for stopping is clinical improvement. Most people dislike taking drugs and will stop as soon as they feel well: this can lead to relapse, particularly in patients prescribed drugs for chronic schizophrenia (see chapter 6) or for recurrent affective disorders (see chapter 7). Among schizophrenics prescribed oral medication 32 per cent were found not to be taking any of their oral medication. The introduction of injectable depot phenothiazines was intended to improve the high defaulter rate, but even with this type of medication a 27 per cent defaulter rate can occur. Depressed patients attending a hospital out-patient department were no better; 44 per cent were found not to be taking their antidepressant medication—even though a considerable number of them had insisted they were doing so. The picture in general practice is more variable; it depends partly on the doctor-patient relationship and partly on the conditions being treated.

It might be thought that the problem of drug defaulting and non-compliance is largely limited to patients who are not resident in hospital. Far from it, careful screening using chromatographic analysis of urine samples has revealed that a considerable proportion, up to 19 per cent in one study, of psychiatric in-patients are not taking their drugs regularly even though they are issued to them by the nursing staff at appropriate times throughout the day.

Lest such findings be thought to be due to vagaries peculiar to psychiatric patients, it should be pointed out that some 50 per cent of patients suffering from rheumatoid arthritis also failed to observe instructions, as did a high proportion of tuberculous patients on anti-tuberculous medication.

Non-pharmacological factors in drug response

Doctor–patient relationship

The doctor–patient relationship not only influences tablet taking but also has a profound effect on the outcome of any course of treatment. First of all, an understanding approach by the doctor will often be sufficient to relieve the patient of his symptoms, particularly where these are the result of worry or tension. In such a situation the benefit attributed to any medication prescribed may be due more to the doctor's manner, and his attitudes towards the drug in question, than to the pharmacological properties of the drug itself. This can lead to an overvaluation of the drug by the doctor and his patient. Even where a true pharmacological effect can be expected this effect may be modified considerably by the doctor–patient relationship. Not unexpectedly, doctors who evince a sceptical attitude towards the drug they are prescribing do not find such drugs nearly as effective as those who prescribe them with enthusiastic optimism. Patients can also influence drug response; any expectations a patient may have about the drug he is receiving can affect the outcome to treatment. Other factors also play a part: males seem to report fewer undesirable side-effects than females, and those of lower intelligence appear to do best overall when treated with psychotropic drugs. This latter finding may be related to the placebo effect.

Placebos

A good definition of what placebos are and how they are used has been formulated by Shapiro:

> A placebo is defined as any therapeutic procedure (or that component of a therapeutic procedure) which is given deliberately to have an effect, or which unknowingly has an effect on the patient's symptom, disease or syndrome, but which is objectively without specific activity for the condition treated. The placebo is also used to describe an adequate control in experimental studies. A placebo effect is defined as the changes produced by placebos.

Many authorities have remarked that a placebo effect was the basis of virtually all medication given before Withering used foxglove in dropsy; Sydenham found Cinchona bark effective in malaria; or Lind noted that fresh fruit was specific for scurvy. Eye of newt and leg of toad are, after all, unlikely to have much in the way of specific activity.

Recent critical interest in the placebo effect has been due in great measure to Beecher, an anaesthetist who observed that soldiers wounded in battle during the Second World War required analgesics less often (in 25 per cent of cases) than surgical patients with far less severe trauma, 80 per cent of whom requested analgesics. He found that a good many of these latter responded to placebo, but whether or not this occurred depended on a number of factors:

1 the nature and quantity of the placebo preparation given
2 the situation and manner in which it was prescribed
3 the social and psychological attributes of the recipient
4 the condition being treated.

1   *The nature and quantity of placebo*   It has been suggested that the shape, size and colour of a tablet can each influence the placebo reaction. Very small tablets (which are by implication very potent) and very large tablets produce a greater effect than those of more moderate size.

Although normal subjects appear relatively unaffected by the colour of the tablet, psychiatric patients presenting with symptoms of anxiety or depression show a differential response to differently coloured pills. In one intriguing study, anxiety symptoms were found to respond most readily to green, whereas depression responded better to yellow tablets. Red tablets were the least effective in both conditions. As might be expected, the greater number of tablets prescribed, the greater the effect within limits; for instance it has been demonstrated that while one 5 mg capsule of amphetamine was superior to a single identical placebo capsule in suppressing subjective hunger, three placebo capsules were better than one active amphetamine capsule.

2   *The situation and manner in which placebo is prescribed*   The profound effect of the doctor–patient relationship in treatment has already been emphasised. Nowhere is this more marked than in placebo treatment. A study which illustrates this point well was carried out on patients presenting with gastrointestinal symptoms associated with diagnosed peptic ulcers. When patients were

prescribed a placebo by a *doctor* who told them that they were getting a new medicine which would bring undoubted relief, 70 per cent of the patients reported definite symptomatic improvement; when prescribed a placebo by a *nurse* who informed them that they were receiving an experimental treatment of unknown efficacy, only 25 per cent benefited. Such variation in outcome in response to the status of the 'healer' and expectation of the patient is undoubtedly the reason why so many more of the seventeenth-century invalids in England preferred being 'touched' by King Charles II, to similar treatment from less exalted figures. It is estimated that this monarch touched over 90,000 patients during his nineteen-year reign.

3 *The social and psychological attributes of the recipient* Although the factors discussed above play a large part in determining the strength of the placebo effect some people appear more likely to react to placebo medication than others. As it would be clinically helpful if such placebo reactors (or responders) could be readily identified many attempts have been made to describe the characteristics which distinguish them from non-reactors. Unfortunately, the findings do not really allow of a clear-cut definition of the placebo reactor. Nevertheless, there appears to be general agreement that the placebo reactor tends to be found more often among younger patients, particularly those of lower intelligence. There is no consistent sex difference, although some investigators have observed more frequent placebo responses in women. Most observers have remarked on the sociability and the apparent desire to please exhibited by the placebo reactor, and a relatively high level of anxiety has also been noted. Although perhaps more anxious in the treatment situation than non-reactors, the placebo reactors do not show widespread neurotic traits and are usually of a stable, rather outgoing personality. It is particularly important to recognise the corollary of this, namely that a patient who is demanding in seeking attention, or particularly complaining, is unlikely to be a placebo reactor, and is thus unlikely to respond to inert medication.

4 *Condition being treated* From studies on the effect of analgesics and placebos on post-operative pain Beecher and Lasagna concluded that placebos are most effective in acute severe stressful situations, being of considerable benefit in post-operative pain,

with some 30 per cent of patients noting relief. They have also been shown to produce symptomatic relief in other acute conditions, including headache, motion sickness, coryza, angina and anxiety.

5 *Mode of action* If placebo acted purely by suggestion then hysterical conversion symptoms might be expected to improve rapidly, but this is one condition where they have proved relatively ineffective. Comparing the effects of repeated placebo administration to those of repeated aspirin administration in a large group of women in labour, Lasagna and his colleagues observed that the time course of efficacy was very similar in both aspirin and placebo; the placebo response was by no means 'all or none'. Similarly the placebo response may persist during the course of several weeks' medication whereas a suggestion response usually disappears within a few days.

Two observations which highlight the complex interaction between patient, the clinical staff and the treatment procedure are (1) morphine addicts, given saline injections instead of morphine, reported no withdrawal symptoms until the saline injections were stopped (2) the substitution of placebo for active medication, without either patients or ward staff being aware of the substitution, in a ward of chronic schizophrenic patients led to no deterioration in behaviour in the majority, and only 29 per cent relapsed; however, when the placebo was stopped and no tablets at all were given the relapse rate immediately increased to 85 per cent.

6 *Side-effects of placebo* In many placebo studies subjective reports of untoward effects often appear, with the following being the most frequent: *sleepiness, dryness of the mouth, headache* and *nausea*. It is obviously necessary to exclude placebo effects as a cause of such symptoms.

Often this may be difficult, as, for instance, when drowsiness follows administration of anxiolytic sedatives, or dryness of the mouth follows treatment with antidepressant drugs.

Occasionally, severe placebo reactions occur; widespread dermatitis, and angioneurotic oedema have been reported. Not only adverse reactions but true dependence to placebo have been noted on at least one occasion with the patient showing all the characteristics of the dependency state, including withdrawal symptoms.

7 *Use of placebo* A placebo may be given wittingly to a patient by a doctor in the hope that it might improve the patient's symptoms and in the knowledge that it is unlikely to make him worse. Few doctors appear to prescribe known inert substances in this manner nowadays, and with the increasing understanding of the psychological factors underlying many symptoms, the indications for such an approach are becoming fewer. It also raises ethical questions which were already being fervently debated at the beginning of the century. One physician went so far as to expostulate: 'Every placebo is a lie. Placebo giving is quackery.'

Much more frequently doctors prescribe medicines of doubtful efficacy, whose therapeutic effect is largely, if not entirely, dependent on a placebo response, in the mistaken belief that the drugs given have a definite specific pharmacological action. Although in many cases this belief is not very firmly held, the mere fact of prescribing relieves both patient and doctor—something is being done. However others have considered this a justifiable psychotherapeutic use of placebo.

Drugs and driving

All centrally acting drugs, if the dose is high enough, have a profound effect on motor skills and reaction time, as well as on the cerebral mechanisms underlying such functions as perception, anticipation and judgment of distance and speed. All these factors are obviously critical in handling complex machinery or driving, where any impairment may well lead to a serious accident. In spite of the considerable potential risk attached to driving while taking psychotropic drugs, relatively little information is available on the subject. This is surprising in view of the ever-increasing number of centrally acting drugs prescribed and the equally expanding volume of traffic on the roads. Those surveys which have been done reveal an alarming lack of concern or even awareness of the problem on the part of most doctors and public authorities. A study in Wales showed that at least 3 per cent of all male drivers and 5 per cent of all female drivers were being prescribed drugs with a central action, the largest single group of drugs being the anxiolytic sedatives. The proportion of drivers being given drugs by doctors is probably even higher in urban areas. In a survey conducted in the UK by the Automobile Association 14 per cent of drivers admitted to having taken some medication in the previous twenty-four hours. Very few had even considered the possible effect such medication might have on their ability to drive, or had been warned by their doctors about it. In the United States some 11 to 16 per cent, and in Canada some 10 to 20 per cent of drivers take drugs regularly, of which at least a quarter are psychoactive. Drug abusers, particularly of the amphetamine type, are especially prone to road traffic accidents (RTA).

Evidence of some association between the ingestion of drugs and road accidents has been obtained in California where 13 per cent of car-drivers involved in fatal single vehicle accidents (i.e. where only the driver of that car was to blame) had measurable quantities of drugs in their circulation. In most cases these were anxiolytic sedatives, neuroleptics and antihistamines, rather than drugs of abuse like cannabis or opiates. However it was considered that the proportion with barbiturates or tranquillisers in their blood was not greater than would be expected in the general population. In Europe the number of drivers involved in road accidents found to have taken drugs, often in conjunction with alcohol, ranges from 10 per cent (Germany) to 16 per cent (Denmark). In a recent study in Norway, blood levels of diazepam were measured in patients hospitalised as a result of RTA and compared to the blood levels of diazepam found in a reference group of drivers attending for routine medical check-up. It was found that those who had been involved in RTA were more likely to have taken diazepam, either alone or in combination with alcohol. Similarly, it has been reported that RTA were more frequent in Japanese taxi drivers who had taken tranquillisers than in those who had not.

Although such statistics provide sufficient cause for concern, there remains the possibility that some drivers, particularly the very anxious, actually drive better when taking moderate doses of anxiolytic sedatives. What we need to know is whether psycho-tropic drugs when given to patients in clinical dosage significantly impair their driving behaviour, and whether RTA are more com-mon among patients taking these drugs than among patients with similar presenting symptoms who have not been taking medication. Unfortunately there is no evidence available on these points; the experimental work that has been done on the effects of anxiolytic sedatives on driving has largely been restricted to normal subjects. Furthermore, most investigations have been limited to measuring the effects of drugs on psychomotor tasks in the laboratory, or driving simulators; these can only provide pointers to the likely effects of drugs on driving, as they bear little relationship to actually driving a car in traffic, which is an extremely complex operation involving attention, perception, motor skills, motivation, and social attitudes. However there have been a few trials of drugs on driving a car in restricted traffic-free areas; the findings have been somewhat equivocal but, in general, there appears to be little impairment of car driving by experienced drivers after ingestion of therapeutic doses of anxiolytic sedatives. Alcohol, on the other hand, significantly impairs driving skills under these conditions, and the combination of psychotropic drugs with alcohol can be particularly dangerous.

Until more is known about the effects that centrally acting drugs have on the driving abilities of patients, the very least that every doctor should do is to warn his patients that their driving might be affected, and urge them to be ultra-cautious, even to the point of not driving, particularly during the first few days of medication, when the unwanted effects are most pronounced; they should also be told firmly to avoid alcohol before driving and to stop driving if they feel at all unwell during a journey.

Suggestions for further reading

National patterns of psychotropic drug prescribing and attitudes

BALTER, M., LEVINE, J., and MANNHEIMER, D. I., 'Cross-national study of the extent of anti-anxiety/sedative drug use', *New England Journal of Medicine*, vol. 290, 1974, pp. 769–74.

DUNLOP, D., 'Abuse of drugs by the public and by doctors', *British Medical Bulletin*, vol. 26, 1970, pp. 236–9.

GREENBLATT, D. J., SHADER, R. I., and KOCH-WESER, J., 'Psychotropic drug use in the Boston Area', *Archives of General Psychiatry*, vol. 32, 1975, pp. 518–21.

MANNHEIMER, D. I., DAVIDSON, S., BALTER, M. B., MELLINGER, G. D., CISIN, I. H., and PARRY, H. J., 'Popular attitudes and beliefs about tranquillisers', *Americal Journal of Psychiatry*, vol. 130, 1973, pp. 1246–53.

PARISH, P., 'The prescribing of psychotropic drugs in general practice', *Journal of the Royal College of General Practitioners*, vol. 21, Supplement no. 4, 1971.

PARISH, P. A., WILLIAMS, W. M., and ELMES, P. C., 'The medical use of psychotropic drugs', *Journal of the Royal College of General Practitioners*, vol. 23, Supplement no. 2, 1973.

PARRY, H. J., BALTER, M. B., MELLINGER, G. D., CISIN, I. H., and MANN-HEIMER, D. I., 'National patterns of psychotherapeutic drug use', *Archives of General Psychiatry*, vol. 28, 1973, pp. 769–83.

WILKS, J. M., 'The use of psychotropic drugs in general practice', *Journal of the Royal College of General Practitioners*, vol. 25, 1975, pp. 731–44.

Drug defaulting

BALLINGER, B. R., SIMPSON, E., and STEWART, M. J., 'An evaluation of a drug administration system in a psychiatric hospital', *British Journal of Psychiatry*, vol. 125, 1974, pp. 202–7.

BLACKWELL, B., 'Treatment adherence', *British Journal of Psychiatry*, vol. 129, 1976, pp. 513–31.

HARE, E. H., and WILCOX, D. R. C., 'Do psychiatric in-patients take their pills ?', *British Journal of Psychiatry*, vol. 113, 1967, pp. 1435–9.

JOHNSON, D. A. W., 'A study of the use of anti-depressant medication in general practice', *British Journal of Psychiatry*, vol. 125, 1974, pp. 186–92.

JOHNSON, D. A. W., and FREEMAN, H., 'Drug defaulting by patients on long-acting phenothiazines', *Psychological Medicine*, vol. 3, 1973, pp. 115–19.

PORTER, A. M. W., 'Drug defaulting in general practice', *British Medical Journal*, vol. 1, 1969, pp. 218–22.

WILCOX, D. R. C., GILLAN, R., and HARE, E. H., 'Do psychiatric out-patients take their drugs ?' *British Medical Journal*, vol. 2, 1965, pp. 790–2.

Non-pharmacological factors in drug response

BEECHER, H. K., 'The powerful placebo', *Journal of the American Medical Association*, vol. 159, 1955, pp. 1602–6.

BLACK, A. A., 'Factors predisposing to a placebo response in new out-patients with anxiety states', *British Journal of Psychiatry*, vol. 112, 1966, pp. 557–67.

HESSBACHER, P. T., RICKELS, K., GORDON, P. E., GRAY, B., MECKELNBURG, R., WELSE, C. C., and VENDERVORT, W. J., 'Setting, patient and doctor effects on drug response in neurotic patients', *Psychopharmacologia*, vol. 18, 1970, pp. 180–208.

HOLLENDER, M. H., 'Observations on the use of the placebo in medical practice', *American Practitioner and Digest of Treatment*, vol. 9, 1958, pp. 214–17.

HONIGFIELD, G., 'Non-specific factors in treatment', *Diseases of the Nervous System*, vol. 25, 1964, pp. 145–56 and pp. 225–39.

HUSSAIN, M. Z., 'Effect of shape of medication in treatment of anxiety states', *British Journal of Psychiatry*, vol. 120, 1972, pp. 507–9.

LASAGNA, L., LATIES, V. G., and DOHAN, J. L., 'Further studies on the "pharmacology" of placebo and administration', *Journal of General Psychiatry*, vol. 20, 1969, pp. 84–8.

LOWINGER, P., and DOBIE, S., 'What makes the placebo work ?' *Archives of General Psychiatry*, vol. 20, 1969, pp. 84–8.

SCHAPIRA, K., MCCLELLAND, H. A., GRIFFITHS, N. R., and NEWELL, D. J., 'Study on the effects of tablet colour in the treatment of anxiety states', *British Medical Journal*, vol. 2, 1970, pp. 446–9.

SHAPIRO, A. K., 'A contribution to a history of the placebo effect', *Behavioural Science*, vol. 5, 1960, pp. 109–35.

WHEATLEY, D., 'Influence of doctors and patients attitudes in the treatment of neurotic illness', *Lancet*, vol. 2. 1967, pp. 1133–5.

Drugs and driving

ASHWORTH, B. M., 'Drugs and driving', *British Journal of Hospital Medicine*, vol. 13, 1975, pp. 201–4.

BØ, O., HAFFNER, J. F. W., LANGARD, O., TRUMPTY, J. H., BREDESEN, J. E., and LUNDE, P. K. M., 'Ethanol and diazepam as causative agents in road accidents', *Proceedings of the 6th International Conference on Alcohol, Drugs and Driving*, Toronto, 1974, pp. 439–48.

BETTS, T. A., CLAYTON, A. B., and MACKAY, G. M., 'Effects of four commonly-used tranquillisers on low-speed driving performance tests', *British Medical Journal*, vol. 4, 1972, pp. 580–4.

GREENBLATT, D. J., and SHADER, R. I., *Benzodiazepines in Clinical Practice*, Raven, New York, 1974, pp. 178–9.

HAVARD, J. D. J., 'Drugs and driving', *British Journal of Hospital Medicine*, vol. 4, 1970, pp. 455–8.

MILNER, G., *Drugs and Driving*, Karger, Basle, 1971.

REES, W. D., 'Psychotropic drugs and the motorist', *Practitioner*, vol. 196, 1966, pp. 704–6.

SEPPALA, T., LINNOILA, M., ELONEN, E., MATTILA, M. J., and MAKI, M., 'Effect of tricyclic anti-depressants and alcohol on psychomotor skills relating to driving', *Clinical Pharmacology and Therapeutics*, vol. 17, 1974, pp. 451–4.

WALLER, J. A., 'Drugs and highway crashes', *Journal of the American Medical Association*, vol. 215, 1971, pp. 1477–82.

Clinical applications

Part II

Schizophrenia 6

Pathogenesis

Schizophrenia, which accounts for one-fifth of all patients currently residing in British hospitals, and for a similar proportion in many other countries, remains one of the least understood conditions in medical practice. In spite of years of painstaking research by teams of highly competent investigators in centres all over the world, almost nothing is known of its basic underlying pathology, or of its aetiology. There are three major obstacles to fundamental research in this area:

1 uncertainty of classification

2 inconsistency in diagnosis

3 inaccessibility of the living human brain to direct observation.

Schizophrenia may present in a number of ways; it is uncertain whether these are varieties of one illness, or several different illnesses, each with its own pathology and aetiology. Comparative studies have revealed that British psychiatrists in particular are more rigorous in making the diagnosis of schizophrenia than their American colleagues. This can lead to discrepancies when workers on one side of the Atlantic compare their findings with those on the other. Nevertheless, there is better agreement on the more florid cases, and certain schizophrenic patients are clearly recognisable as such whatever their cultural background. Probably the most significant barrier to advancement is the practical and ethical problem of examining the human brain directly. The biochemical and physiological changes within the depths of the brain, which probably underlie the strange and bewildering array of symptoms characteristic of this illness, remain largely inaccessible to direct examination. The majority of studies in this field have therefore been limited to the relatively crude approach of examining body fluids, particularly blood and urine, in the hope of finding alterations in them which might afford a clue to pathogenesis. Recently psychopharmacological investigations in men as well as in laboratory animals have led to a considerable increase in our understanding of this baffling condition.

Biochemical theories of schizophrenia

Although there is no certainty regarding the biochemical basis of schizophrenia, a number of theories have been put forward: of these the most widely accepted is the dopamine hypothesis.

Dopamine hypothesis

An abnormality of the dopamine (DA) pathways within the brain has been implicated as a pathogenic factor in schizophrenia for two main reasons: first, all known effective neuroleptic compounds block dopamine receptors both *in vivo* and *in vitro*; second, amphetamine, which in high dosage can produce a paranoid psychosis closely resembling schizophrenia, probably acts in the CNS by releasing dopamine and noradrenaline (NA) from nerve terminals. As the dextro-isomer of amphetamine is only slightly more effective than the laevo-isomer in producing psychosis, it is thought that the psychosis is DA rather than NA mediated. Amphetamine psychosis is also ameliorated by neuroleptics (i.e. DA receptor blocking drugs), and naturally occurring psychosis is made worse by amphetamine and by methylphenidate.

However it would be an oversimplification to suggest that schizophrenia in all its varied forms is but a reflection of a generalised overactivity within DA pathways, or of a supersensitivity of DA receptors throughout the brain. Examination of the CSF of schizophrenic patients has failed to reveal any significant increase in the metabolites of DA; this would argue against any generalised increase of DA activity in the acute condition. However on recovery, homovanillic acid (the metabolite of DA) may fall sharply.

It should be remembered (see chapter 2) that there are at least four distinct DA pathways within the brain: the nigro-striatal which is concerned with motor co-ordination and which is affected in Parkinson's disease; the medullary pathway which is possibly identical with the vomiting centre; the hypothalamic-pituitary pathway which affects the release of the hormone prolactin from the pituitary (DA is thought to be an inhibitor of prolactin release by the pituitary); the mesolimbic pathway, which has extensions to the cortex. It is this mesolimbic pathway which is believed to be the one most likely to be involved in schizophrenia.

Other evidence against a general abnormality of brain DA being a causal factor in schizophrenia is the finding that prolactin levels are not raised in patients with the illness; furthermore, parkinsonism, which is a reflection of DA insufficiency within the nigro-striatal system, can co-exist with schizophrenia. Thus schizophrenia can hardly be due to a generalised excess DA activity, although it does not rule out a more localised overactivity of DA, perhaps in the mesolimbic system. In keeping with such a view is the observation that the relative potency of neuroleptics as anti-psychotic agents in man is closely reflected by their relative potency as DA receptor blockers in the limbic system, but not in the nigro-striatal system of laboratory animals. It would appear that abnormality of DA, either in terms of metabolism, or release, or of the receptors within the mesolimbic system of the brain is associated with schizophrenia; lesions of this system, such as occur in some cases of temporal lope epilepsy, can lead to a syndrome resembling schizophrenia. But before we can assume that, because neuroleptics act as DA receptor blockers, schizophrenia is due to over-activity in one or more DA systems within the brain, we must consider other alternatives. Schizophrenia may be the result of an imbalance between more than one neurotransmitter system. A hint that this might be so is provided by the finding that physostigmine, a centrally active cholinesterase inhibitor (which leads to excess acetylcholine at the synapse due to reduced breakdown by cholinesterase), can protect against methylphenidate-induced exacerbation of schizophrenia, without being effective against the underlying condition. It may be that the DA mesolimbic pathway is involved in arousal which in turn affects some other, as yet unknown, part of the brain in which the primary lesion lies. If this were true the action of the neuroleptics would be to reduce central arousal, thereby secondarily affecting this, as yet hypothetical, primary system; these drugs would not, however, directly affect the fundamental lesion. Such a view would be consistent with the failure of a proportion of patients with schizophrenia to improve on medication with neuroleptic drugs.

Other possible imbalances between neurotransmitters have been suggested: these include an increase in DA relative to NA, and an increase of DA relative to 5-hydroxytryptamine (5HT). This latter suggestion would also involve the concept of arousal, as 5HT is generally believed to be concerned in the regulation of sleep and waking; with lowered 5HT reducing sleep and increasing arousal. Thus elevation of DA activity and reduction of 5HT activity could act synergistically to increase arousal and thereby exacerbate the underlying schizophrenic syndrome.

We would conclude that, while it would appear that DA is involved in the pathogenesis of schizophrenia in some way in some patients, the mechanism of its involvement remains to be determined.

Transmethylation hypothesis

Mescaline, a hallucinogenic compound used in certain religious rites in Mexico (see chapter 1), was noted to be an ortho-methylated derivative of dopamine. From this observation came the suggestion that schizophrenia might itself be due to a disturbance of transmethylation of neurotransmitter substances within the brain leading to the production of hallucinogens. If this were true, then reduction of such methylated derivatives should improve the condition. To this end nicotinic acid and nicotinamide were put forward as potential methyl acceptors, that is compounds which would divert methyl groups from neurotransmitters, thereby lessening the likelihood of formation of possible hallucinogenic substances within the brain.

Both nicotinic acid and nicotinamide, even in very high dosage, have proved ineffective in alleviating symptoms of schizophrenia. However, this result does not nullify the transmethylation hypothesis as it has subsequently been shown that these substances would not in fact compete with methylation processes in the CNS.

Looking at the problem another way, the administration of the methyl donor methionine together with a monoamine oxidase inhibitor appeared to exacerbate the clinical state in a proportion of patients suffering from schizophrenia: normal subjects given similar doses of methionine showed no psychotic effect. Other studies indicated that a substance present in the brain, 5 methyltetrahydrofolic acid (MTHF), could act as a methyl donor for phenylethylamines (such as DA and NA) and for indoleamines (such as 5HT) to produce compounds with marked hallucinogenic properties (such as demethyltryptamine (DMT) and 5-methoxy— N, N—dimethyltryptamine (OMB). This view is not universally accepted; an alternative proposition is that MTHF provides methyl groups to form S-adenosylethionine which in turn acts as a methyldonor to DA.

Although the necessary enzymes and precursors may be present in the brain for such substances to be formed, the evidence to date suggests that neither DMT or OMB is significantly different in the CSF of schizophrenics as compared to normal control subjects. In any case the original premise on which the transmethylation hypothesis is based appears somewhat unlikely in that mescaline, although a hallucinogen, does not produce symptoms reminiscent of schizophrenia in the same way that amphetamine does. Thus the levels of hallucinogenic substances within the brain may have very little to do with the biochemical basis of the illness or illnesses called schizophrenia.

Psychopathology

It is perhaps not surprising that no single theory of schizophrenia has obtained universal acceptance when one considers that there are a number of sub-types of the illness, and that its manifestations can vary considerably from patient to patient depending on the sub-type present, the cultural background and the pre-morbid personality. There are four main areas of psychological function which may be disturbed in schizophrenia, and correspondingly four varieties of the condition. The areas of malfunction involve perception, thought processes, emotional responsiveness, and motor activity.

Perceptual disorders

The most frequent of the perceptual disorders are auditory hallucinations (hearing voices). Patients can usually hear involved conversations between two or more voices (phonemes) which frequently make disparaging references to the patient, referring to him in the third person. Sometimes the voices will give the patient orders thereby producing unpredictable behaviour. Other hallucinations (i.e. perceptions without stimuli) can occur, such as sensations of electricity in the skin (tactile hallucinations) and strange smells or tastes (olfactory and gustatory hallucinations). Visual hallucinations are rare in schizophrenia, although characteristic of hallucinogenic drug-induced states. Auditory hallucinations also occur in chronic alcohol poisoning and acute amphetamine intoxication, implying a definite organic basis for their origin.

Thought disorder

Many schizophrenic patients, although not lacking in intelligence, are unable to put their thoughts together in a comprehensible fashion. This leads to a failure by the observer to grasp exactly what it is the patient is saying although the individual words and phrases appear to be quite normal. It is this peculiar lack of understandability of the train of thought which, when present, is pathognomonic of schizophrenia. Thought disorder of the schizophrenic type does not occur in any other mental illness and is not produced by any of the hallucinogenic drugs. Thus, hypotheses of schizophrenia based solely on a hallucinogenic drug model are unlikely to provide a complete answer to the problem of understanding the biochemical basis of the illness.

As well as having a disordered way of thinking (disorder of form), schizophrenic patients frequently believe quite irrationally that they are being persecuted, pursued or spied upon (paranoid delusions). Such delusions (or disorders of content) may exist without any disorder of form being present. Paranoid delusions, like auditory hallucinations, may also occur in amphetamine intoxication and in acute confusional states (see chapter 9). Other disorders of thought content include ideas that messages are being given to the patient on the radio or in the newspapers (ideas of reference) and the feeling that he is being controlled by an outside influence (passivity feelings).

Emotional disturbance

Characteristically, schizophrenic patients appear lacking in emotional responsiveness, presenting a blank, disinterested facial appearance (emotional 'flattening'); sometimes they may respond quite unexpectedly by laughing in the wrong places, or giggling to themselves (incongruity of affect); both these phenomena are particularly prevalent in the hebephrenic and simple forms of schizophrenia.

Motor behaviour

Certain patients gradually become less and less active, lapsing eventually into an apparently stuporous state (catatonia). This state may be interrupted by an outburst of violent activity (catatonic excitement) which ends as suddenly as it begins. Although extreme catatonia is now rare, less severe forms of inactivity and lack of drive are not uncommon.

Types of schizophrenia

Schizophrenia has been classified largely on the basis of the predominant symptoms or group of symptoms present. Whether or not the different types each have different aetiology and pathogenesis is not known.

1 *Paranoid schizophrenia* This is usually of acute onset and is the most common form in the elderly. Auditory hallucinations and paranoid delusions dominate the clinical picture. This form is of good prognosis and the most responsive to neuroleptic drugs.

2 *Hebephrenic schizophrenia* This usually comes on gradually and is of less favourable prognosis. It is more common in adolescents and young adults. Incongruity of affect and schizophrenic thought disorder are the most prominent symptoms.

3 *Catatonic schizophrenia* This is the least common, usually having an acute onset in adolescence, and is characterised by catatonic motor symptoms (see above) with underlying thought disorder and delusions.

4 *Simple schizophrenia* This manifests as a gradual withdrawal from all social activity and a corresponding lack of motivation and drive. Flattening of affect is a feature, and thought disorder may be present.

Pharmacology of neuroleptic drugs

The drugs used in the treatment of schizophrenia were originally referred to as neuroleptics because of their ability to produce a state of 'neurolepsis' or calm indifference without loss of consciousness. They may be subdivided into several groups. These include rauwolfia alkaloids, phenothiazines, thioxanthenes, indole derivatives, butyrophenones and diphenylbutylpiperidines.

Rauwolfia alkaloids

Extracts of plants of the rauwolfia variety have been used in Asia for centuries for a number of conditions, including insanity and hypertension, but it was only some twenty years ago that the alkaloid reserpine was isolated and introduced into clinical medicine.

The calming effects of reserpine are probably related to its ability to deplete the brain of monoamine stores. Its therapeutic ratio is relatively narrow, however, and administration of higher doses may result in: mental depression which may be suicidal, extrapyramidal disorders with parkinsonism, choreoathetosis and ataxia (probably due to dopamine depletion in the basal ganglia), and finally to central respiratory depression and death. Diarrhoea, nasal stuffiness, fluid retention with cardiac failure and endocrine disorders, such as amenorrhoea, gynaecomastia and impairment of sexual function, can also occur. Increased gastric secretion can lead to reactivation of a peptic ulcer or to the development of new ulcers, possibly complicated by haemorrhage and perforation. In addition, the depletion of pressor substances resulting from reserpine administration may cause prolonged hypotension and bradycardia during the stress of anaesthesia and surgery.

Reserpine is readily absorbed from the gastrointestinal tract and from parenteral sites of injection. There are a variety of metabolites which are only slowly eliminated from the body. Reserpine appears to be taken up rapidly by lipid-containing tissues throughout the body, and is cumulative in action, so that any change in dosage should be carried out slowly and cautiously. It has been superseded almost entirely by the phenothiazines in the treatment of schizophrenia.

Phenothiazines

The discovery that the phenothiazine derivative promethazine possesses sedative and antihistamine actively encouraged the synthesis of other compounds in this group. Chlorpromazine, synthesised in 1950, was soon found to have pronounced calmative effects on disturbed psychotic patients. Since then it has come to be the standard compound against which other substances have been compared. Phenothiazines have a large number of pharmacological properties, and minor changes in their molecular structure may profoundly influence their therapeutic activity and the severity of unwanted effects, particularly the incidence of extrapyramidal reactions. All drugs in this group have in common the pheno-thiazine nucleus:

Derivatives are usually formed by substitution at positions R_1 and R_2. The side chains at R_1 may be classified into three groups: (i) dimethylaminopropyl (aliphatic) (ii) piperazine (iii) piperidine. The substitutions at R_2 include halogens, methoxy, acetyl, thio-methyl, and other organic radicals. Compounds such as promazine, which is unsubstituted at position R_2, are very much less active pharmacologically than derivatives with chloro- or trifluoromethyl substitutions at that position, such as chlorpromazine or trifluo-promazine; this variation in pharmacological effect has been related to the stoichiometric configuration of the molecule; Snyder talks of the compounds being 'sculpted' to fit the DA receptor where they act to block transmission by DA. It also appears that the different substituents on the phenothiazine ring determine the site of action by altering the distribution of the drug, the more potent compounds having substituents which increase their lipid solubility and facilitate their transport into the brain. Their pharmacological actions depend on the electronic nature of the phenothiazine ring and involve electron donation in charge-transfer reactions.

1 *Neurochemical action* Phenothiazine compounds act by block-ing dopamine receptors in all four dopaminergic systems of the brain. After the postsynaptic DA receptors have been blocked by these drugs there is a feedback mechanism whereby the presynaptic neurone releases more DA to overcome the blockade; this in turn increases the production and turnover of DA with a corresponding increase in its metabolites. In fact, the finding of such an increase in the metabolites of dopamine, led Carlsson to suggest that phenothiazine drugs might act as DA receptor blockers. Reduction of this compensatory DA synthesis, as occurs after blocking the enzyme tyrosine hydroxylase with alpha-methylparatyrosine, en-hances the anti-psychotic activity of chlorpromazine, thus confirm-ing that it is DA receptor blockade which is the basis of the

therapeutic action of chlorpromazine. The relative potency of the various phenothiazine compounds is not the same at all sites. For example, thioridazine, which has a piperidine side chain, is less effective than a clinically equivalent dose of chlorpromazine, which has an aliphatic side chain, on increasing DA metabolism in the nigro-striatal system; chlorpromazine in turn has less effect than a clinically equivalent dose of fluphenazine, which has a piperazine side-chain. This finding is in keeping with the greater tendency of the piperazine phenothiazines to produce extrapyramidal symptoms. Drugs such as thioridazine, which are less likely to produce extrapyramidal symptoms, and which have correspondingly less effect of DA turnover in the striatum, have an in-built anticholinergic action. It is thought that DA neurones in the striatum inhibit acetylcholine neurones, which normally activiate gamma amino butyric acid (GABA) neurones. These GABA neurones, in turn, inhibit the DA neurones, see Figure 4. If the action of acetylcholine is blocked at the same time as the DA receptor, then the effects on the motor system are cancelled out, whereas if the acetylcholine system is freed from dopaminergic inhibition, then extrapyramidal symptoms emerge.

In the mesolimbic system, in contrast to what happens in the striatum, the three drugs, thioridazine, chlorpromazine and fluphenazine have similar effects on dopamine turnover when given in clinically equivalent dosage. This finding is consistent with the view that the efficacy of these drugs on schizophrenia is more closely related to a possible action within the mesolimbic system than elsewhere in the brain.

The phenothiazines are potent antiemetic drugs, preventing vomiting produced by other drugs such as apomorphine which stimulate the dopaminergic chemoreceptor trigger zone. An action on neighbouring medullary areas may be responsible for their usefulness in the control of persistent hiccough.

There is at least one other dopaminergic system on which phenothiazines act; that is the hypothalmic pituitary portal pathway which controls the release of prolactin from the pituitary. Dopamine inhibits the release of prolactin so that DA receptor blocking drugs, such as phenothiazines, by preventing this DA mediated inhibition, allow more prolactin to be released into the circulation, thus raising the serum prolactin level. It has recently been found that if the prolactin level rises above 30 ng/ml two hours after the administration of chlorpromazine, extrapyramidal

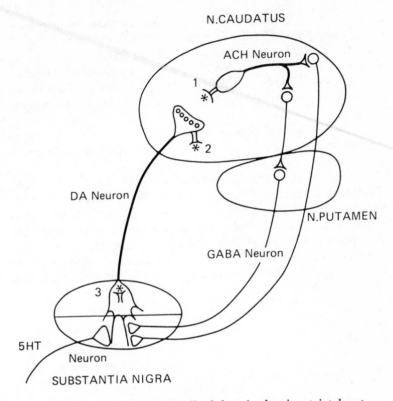

Figure 4   *The neurochemical feedback loop in the nigrostriatal system* (from J. Glowinski, in *Biology of the Major Psychoses*, ed. D. X. Freed- man, Raven Press, New York, 1975)

symptoms are likely to follow. Furthermore there appears to be a significant correlation between the plasma levels of prolactin and of chlorpromazine. The plasma prolactin level promises to afford a useful index of central dopaminergic blockade. Raised prolactin levels can produce galactorrhoea in women and gynaecomastia in men (see below). In addition to their DA receptor blocking activity the phenothiazines have a variable anticholinergic activity (see above) and weak to moderate antihistamine and anti-5HT activity.

2   *Pharmacokinetics*   Chlorpromazine, which has been the most widely studied of the phenothiazines, is readily absorbed from the gastrointestinal tract and from intra-muscular injection sites, with a peak blood level occurring some 1·5 to 3 hours after oral

97

administration. Sometimes absorption may be poor, with consequently low plasma levels. Distribution within the body is rapid, with the highest concentrations occurring in the lungs, liver, adrenal glands and spleen. Within the brain there would appear to be a selective distribution, with the highest concentration being found in the hypothalmus, basal ganglia, thalamus and hippocampus.

As yet no optimal plasma level for chlorpromazine has been established although the ratio of active metabolites to the more inert ones may be of some importance.

Chlorpromazine can be metabolised in a number of ways, illustrated in Figure 5. Of the metabolites the 7-hydroxy derivative is pharmacologically active whereas the sulphoxide is not; consequently if there is a relatively large proportion of sulphoxide therapeutic response is less. Chlorpromazine has an enzyme-inducing effect which in turn can effect the concentration in the body of other compounds (see chapter 3 for a further discussion of this point).

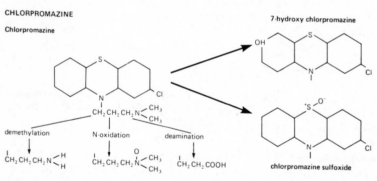

Figure 5 *The metabolic pathways of chlorpromazine*

Chlorpromazine has a plasma half-life of some six hours; however, it can remain bound to the tissues for very long periods, and metabolites may continue to be excreted for up to six months after the patient has stopped taking it.

3 *Interaction with other drugs* Phenothiazines enhance the central depressant effects of many other drugs including barbiturates and alcohol. They also potentiate the analgesic effect of the

narcotic analgesic drugs; this may be of therapeutic value in patients with severe pain, particularly where it results from neoplastic diseases and is accompanied by marked anxiety.

While they only possess a weak anticholinergic activity themselves, when combined with an anticholinergic compound prescribed to relieve parkinsonian side-effects, an atropine-type psychosis can occur due to the additive atropine-like activity.

Thioxanthenes

In these compounds the nitrogen in the central ring of the phenothiazine is replaced by carbon. The analogues thus formed appear to be no more effective than their phenothiazine progenitors.

Butyrophenones

Although the butyrophenone compounds are structurally distinct from the phenothiazines they share many of their pharmacological properties. Like the phenothiazines they cause accumulation of O-methylated metabolites of dopamine and noradrenaline within the brain, suggesting that they also block dopamine and noradrenaline receptors, thus causing compensatory activity of central neurones with monoamine transmitter release. In the peripheral autonomic nervous system butyrophenones such as haloperidol and trifluperidol selectively block dopamine receptors in the renal and mesenteric vascular beds, and it may be that a similar selectivity of action occurs in the central nervous system.

The butyrophenones are also potent antiemetic drugs, suppressing activity of the chemoreceptor trigger zone, and they produce extrapyramidal disorders similar to those accompanying phenothiazine medication. They also potentiate the sedative effects of alcohol, analgesics, anaesthetics and barbiturate drugs, and transient orthostatic hypotension can occur, due to peripheral adrenergic receptor blockade.

Diphenylbutylpiperidines

These compounds, derived from the butyrophenones, have a more prolonged duration of action. They would also seem to have a more specific dopamine receptor blocking action. Two members of this group are in clinical use, pimozide, which can be given orally on a daily basis, and fluspiriline, which requires to be administered intramuscularly, a single injection of which has an effective action of one week.

Penfluridol, a drug which is still under investigation, is another long acting derivative which appears to be clinically effective when given by mouth at weekly intervals.

Other drugs

Tetrabenazine This is a synthetic benzoquinolizine which retains some of the structural features of reserpine and has an identical pharmacology. It depletes the brain of its monoamine stores and this is probably the basis of its sedative and antipsychotic effects. Mental depression and extrapyramidal reactions commonly occur. Its dopamine depleting property is said to be useful in the management of tardive dyskinesia.

Certain indole derivatives, such as *oxypertine* and *molindone* appear to possess antipsychotic properties. Other dibenzyl structures including *clozapine* and *metiapine* have similar effects with less tendency to produce parkinsonian symptoms.

Drug treatment

Acute schizophrenia

An acute schizophrenic episode frequently presents with obvious delusory ideas, accompanied by auditory hallucinations. In addition there may be frank thought disorder with ideas of reference, ideas of influence and passivity feelings. Such a situation, whether arising for the first time, or resulting from a relapse in a patient who has had a similar illness in the past, calls for energetic medication with one of the neuroleptic drugs. This can be done either on an in-patient or an out-patient basis, although generally speaking the majority of patients suffering from acute schizophrenia will require in-patient treatment for a short time, particularly if they are disturbed in their behaviour.

1 *Initial control* Once the diagnosis of acute schizophrenia has been made, the next step is to decide on the choice of medication and the route of administration. If, as is usually the case, there is a certain amount of motor excitement, arising perhaps out of the patient's delusional fears, administration of a neuroleptic with sedative effects would be advisable. A phenothiazine with an

aliphatic side-chain such as chlorpromazine is particularly suitable. It is difficult to be dogmatic about dosage but the following guidelines are suggested:

(i) In the case of a healthy male patient under the age of sixty, up to 300 mg of the drug may be given as a starting dose. This can be repeated as necessary up to four times in twenty-four hours for the first few days. In most cases it is usually possible to reduce the dosage to between 100 and 200 mg twice or four times daily within a short time. The physician will need to be guided on the one hand by the amount by which disturbed behaviour has been reduced and on the other hand by the degree of somnolence produced by the medication. It may be that the first dose produces so much drowsiness that the dosage can be sharply reduced almost immediately. Sometimes, however, even 300 mg of chlorpromazine proves inadequate to reduce the acute disturbance sufficiently and an even higher dosage may be required. In many cases with frank behaviour disturbance, the oral route is not possible and the drug has to be given intramuscularly. The dosage of chlorpromazine would be the same, but the addition of an equal amount of amylobarbitone sodium often produces a more satisfactory effect. Intramuscular administration is rarely required after the first 24–48 hours, as by then the patient has usually become sufficiently cooperative to take his drugs by mouth.

(ii) A healthy woman under the age of sixty should be given up to 200 mg chlorpromazine as a starting dose, otherwise the initial drug treatment is as outlined for a healthy male.

(iii) A patient who is known to be in frail physical health, or anyone over the age of sixty, should not be given more than 100 mg chlorpromazine in the first instance. Particular care should be taken in patients with cardiovascular abnormalities lest drug-induced hypotension should embarrass their circulation yet further. Similarly those with a known history of liver disease should be treated cautiously as they are often particularly sensitive to the central effects of phenothiazine compounds.

Haloperidol (Haldol, Serenace) may be substituted for chlorpromazine either when an injection is required or when given orally. Haloperidol is approximately fifty to one hundred times more potent than chlorpromazine, thus each milligram of haloperidol is equivalent to between 50 and 100 mg of chlorpromazine.

It is claimed that haloperidol acts rather more quickly and produces less sedation than chlorpromazine, with less risk of hypertension occurring.

2 *Amelioration of schizophrenic symptoms* Once control of disturbed behaviour has been achieved the next step is to decide upon the most suitable treatment of the particular symptom complex present in the individual case. The symptoms most responsive to neuroleptic medication are paranoid delusions and auditory hallucinations; thought disorder, apathy and abnormalities of emotional response are less likely to improve so gratifyingly.

There is a bewildering choice of drugs available, all of which have been claimed to be useful in the management of schizophrenia. These include some ten phenothiazine compounds, four thioxanthene derivatives, at least three butyrophenones and three members of the closely related diphenylbutylpiperidines, plus a number of others (see Table 6).

Several well-conducted large-scale clinical trials have failed to reveal any significant differences in overall efficacy between one neuroleptic phenothiazine and another. Furthermore, although it had been suggested that those phenothiazine drugs with piperazine side-chains (e.g. trifluoperazine and fluphenazine) were more effective than the aliphatic phenothiazines (e.g. chlorpromazine) in stimulating apathetic schizophrenic patients into activity, the evidence obtained from the clinical trials fails to support this suggestion. The choice of drug depends more upon the side-effects produced, which vary from drug to drug, and upon the frequency of dosage required.

Chlorpromazine remains the standard medication in schizophrenia against which other treatments must be measured. It has been repeatedly shown to be more effective in schizophrenia than an inert placebo or an anxiolytic sedative such as phenobarbitone. It is also better than the antihistamine compound promethazine from which it was originally derived. With chlorpromazine over 60 per cent of patients with acute schizophrenic symptoms can be expected to improve significantly within a matter of weeks. The dosage of chlorpromazine required to achieve this varies considerably from case to case but is rarely less than 100 mg three times a day and may be as high as 300 mg four times daily. Once a steady state has been achieved it may be possible to reduce the dose by half without a recrudescence of symptoms. The drawbacks of chlorpromazine are its sedative effects and tendency to produce extrapyramidal symptoms (see below), together with the possibility of cholestatic jaundice, although the incidence of this seems to be falling. If over-sedation proves a problem in management with chlorpromazine then one of the piperazine compounds such as tri-fluoperazine (Stelazine) 5–10 mg or fluphenazine (Moditen, Pro-lixin) 2·5–5 mg three times daily may be tried. While they are certainly less sedating, they produce rather more extrapyramidal symptoms (see below). In contrast thioridazine (Melleril), 100–200 mg three times daily is the least likely of all the phenothiazines to cause such unwanted effects, but it, too, has its drawbacks. It is as sedative as chlorpromazine and is rather more likely to produce hypotension. In addition it interferes with ejaculation in men and may consequently prove unacceptable to many male patients if given over a period longer than a month or two, in addition there is the risk of producing retinal pigmentation.

Neither the thioxanthene derivatives nor the butyrophenones appear to have any advantage over the phenothiazines in the management of schizophrenia. The newer compounds in the di-phenylbutylpiperidine group may prove to be more useful. Pimozide (Orap) requires only once daily administration at a dose of 4 to 40 mg per day. This is not only an advantage to the nurses in a busy psychiatric ward, but it also means that the prescribed dosage is more likely to be taken by the patient at home if he has to remember to take his pills only once during the day instead of three times. In this connection, however, it has recently been suggested that phenothiazine medication need only be given twice daily at most, once initial control has been obtained. Fluspiriline (Redep-tin) reduces the frequency of administration required to weekly, but it has to be given intramuscularly, and this may be less accept-able in some patients.

3 *Longer term medication*   How long should one go on treating an acute episode of schizophrenia ? There is no really clear-cut answer possible, for that depends on the presenting illness. If the episode is the first manifestation of schizophrenia in a particular patient of a previously good personality, and if there was no emotional abnormality during the illness, which itself was of acute onset and short duration, then the chances are that longer-term medication will not prove necessary. In a recent study it was found that among a group of such patients given no further medication after

discharge from hospital the relapse rate was just over 25 per cent. When these criteria were not met, the relapse rate without further drug treatment among those who had responded reasonably well to treatment in the acute phase was over 80 per cent. In contrast, long-term treatment in this second group reduced the relapse rate to 33 per cent. Thus some patients will recover completely from acute schizophrenia and require no further drug treatment for the time being, whereas other patients never fully recover in the sense that they can remain symptom-free without medication. This latter group is often referred to as suffering from chronic schizophrenia, and management of this condition raises problems of its own.

Chronic schizophrenia

If after a first attack of schizophrenia the patient relapses shortly after his medication is stopped then it is likely that he is suffering from the chronic form of the condition and will require continuous medication for years, if not for life. While this need for long-term treatment may well be recognised by the medical advisers concerned with treatment, it is frequently not accepted by the patient. Consequent failure to take the medication leads to recrudescence of symptoms with readmission; in fact the most common cause for readmission to hospital is a relapse following failure to take the drugs prescribed.

As in the case of acute schizophrenia, no one neuroleptic drug stands out from the rest in terms of efficacy, provided the drug is taken. Several investigations have revealed how inconstant and unreliable many patients are in their medication. They stop it either because they feel well and can see no point in continuing, or because the side-effects are sufficiently unpleasant to deter them from persevering. Although such behaviour is by no means confined to schizophrenics (see chapter 5), it creates particularly severe management problems in them. What is required is some way of ensuring that schizophrenic patients take their medication for as long as is considered necessary. The introduction of the long-acting fluphenazine compounds fluphenazine enanthate (Moditen enanthate) and fluphenazine decanoate (Modecate) given by intramuscular injection every one to four weeks has gone a long way to meeting this requirement.

If, however, a patient is known to be reliable in taking oral medication, then there is no need to change his treatment regime to intramuscular injections. Only when it is considered unlikely that a particular patient is going to take his tablets conscientiously outside hospital is it advisable to stabilise him on a programme of fluphenazine injections before he is discharged. A test dose of 12·5 mg (0·5 ml) is usually given. If after a week no untoward reaction has occurred then a dose of 25 mg (1·0 ml) can be given. The administration requires some care: the drug must be given by deep intramuscular injection, preferably into the gluteal region. The most common untoward reaction is the development of extra-pyramidal symptoms (see below) which usually manifest themselves two to eight days after the injection. In addition, certain patients can become severely depressed during treatment with intramuscular long-acting fluphenazine; when this occurs, treatment with tricyclic antidepressant drugs as for depressive illness (see chapter 10) may help.

Flupenthixol decanoate (Depixol) 20–40 mg every one to three weeks is said not to cause depression; on the contrary, a definite antidepressant activity has been remarked upon by some observers.

Patients are usually asked to attend special clinics to receive their regular injections. This not only allows an efficient routine to be adopted by the patients and the nursing staff administering the fluphenazine injections, but it makes it easy to spot when a patient fails to attend. In that case he can either be asked to come up for his injection at another time, or, failing that, he can be visited in his home by a nurse who can give him the long-acting fluphenazine injection there and then. The adoption of such a treatment programme for patients with chronic schizophrenia discharged into the community has been shown to reduce the relapse rate dramatically. There are other injectable long-acting neuroleptics, such as fluspirilene, but they do not appear to possess any added advantages.

More recently a long-acting oral compound, penfluridol, has been developed. It is a member of the diphenylbutylpiperidine group of drugs. Preliminary reports suggest that oral administration once a week of penfluridol in a dose of 10–40 mg can maintain patients symptom-free. Pimozide (Orap) in a daily oral dose of 8 mg appears to be at least as effective as regular depot injections of fluphenazine.

The maintenance therapy of those chronic schizophrenic patients whose symptoms do not remit sufficiently for them to live outside hospital is not so difficult to control and supervise. Here the problem may be one of unnecessarily prolonged medication rather than its absence. These patients remain incapable of leading an independent life in spite of adequate neuroleptic treatment. In many cases stopping their drug does not lead to any deterioration in their condition; on the contrary there may be marked improvement associated with lessening of extrapyramidal symptoms. Even in those patients in whom continued medication is shown to be of benefit, a reduction in dosage may be achieved. Therefore, it is advisable to review from time to time the medication of all long-term in-patients receiving continuous neuroleptic therapy.

Beta-adrenergic receptor blocking drugs in schizophrenia

A number of recently published, uncontrolled reports have suggested that the beta adrenergic receptor blocking drug propranolol (Inderal), when given in high dosage (0·5 to 1·5 g a day) to patients with either acute or chronic schizophrenia, has produced significant improvement in a substantial number.

These reports await confirmation by double blind clinical trial before their findings can be finally accepted. Until then the use of propranolol in schizophrenia must remain experimental.

Unwanted effects of neuroleptic drugs

Extrapyramidal symptoms

These can be considered under four headings:

The first three are relatively acute, they are also clearly dose-dependent and disappear when medication ceases. The fourth group appears often to be irreversible, sometimes even getting worse after neuroleptic treatment has ceased.

Such reactions occur in up to 40 per cent of patients treated with phenothiazines, being more common with those compounds having a piperazine side-chain. They are equally frequent with butyrophenone medication.

1 *Pseudo-parkinsonism* The clinical picture mimics idiopathic parkinsonism very closely, with a general stiffening of the limbs, lack of facial expression, characteristic coarse tremor of the hands and head at rest, plus sialorrhoea and seborrhoea. This may even go on to a complete seizing up with a virtual absence of movement. Chlorpromazine is particularly prone to produce this syndrome.

2 *Akathisia* This condition of restlessness causes great distress to the patient, who feels he cannot keep still. This leads him to

fidget continuously, shuffling up and down, or rocking his body backwards and forwards. This syndrome occurs most often with piperazine phenothiazines.

3 *Acute dyskinesias* These are more acute reactions, of which the oculogyric crisis is probably the best known. It begins with a fixed stare which then gives way to a turning upwards of the eyes followed by hyperextension of the neck and opening of the mouth. The attack may last several hours before subsiding spontaneously. The dyskinesic reactions can also involve the trunk or limb, producing grotesque postures or writhing movements, which are extremely distressing.

4 *Chronic tardive dyskinesia* This condition is characterised by virtually continuous movements of the head and tongue and certain postural changes. They may persist for years after all neuroleptic medication has been stopped. While they were originally thought to be particularly prevalent in patients with brain damage who had received phenothiazine medication in high dosage for years, this has now been shown not to be necessarily true. In fact some doubt has even been cast on the relationship to phenothiazines, as in one series at least 25 per cent of the patients with this condition had never received any neuroleptic drug. It is important to recognise this complication early, and to take appropriate action as soon as possible (see below).

The management of unwanted drug effects

Extrapyramidal reactions

The first step in the management of drug-induced pseudoparkinsonism and akathisia is to stop the drug temporarily or sharply reduced the dose. Many patients will not deteriorate if their medication stops for a few days, particularly if they have been receiving it for several weeks. This measure, together with the administration of an anti-parkinsonian drug is usually sufficient. Of those available benzhexol (Artane) 2–4 mg, procyclidine (Kemadrine) 5–10 mg, orphenadrine (Disipal) 50–100 mg, and methixene (Tremonil) 5–10 mg three times daily would appear to be equally effective; Contrary to the situation in idiopathic parkinsonism, levodopa makes schizophrenic patients with phenothiazine-induced parkinsonism worse. However, a newer type of anti-parkinsonian agent, amantadine (which releases dopamine from neuronal stores), when given in a dose of 100–200 mg per day, may prove to be useful; but thus far clinical trials have not established its efficacy in drug-induced parkinsonism.

Acute dyskinesia responds best to parenteral procyclidine (Kemedrine) 5–10 mg or biperiden (Akineton) 2–5 mg given either by slow intravenous injection or intramuscularly. Intravenous diazepam at a dose of 10 mg has also been found to be effective.

We do not recommend the routine administration of anti-parkinsonian agents to all patients receiving neuroleptics. Not only may they be unnecessary, but also they produce other unwanted effects of their own, particularly anticholergenic symptoms which exacerbate the autonomic actions produced by the phenothiazines themselves.

Persistent chronic dyskinesia is much more resistant to treatment, although there are recent reports that tetrabenazine 25 mg three to four times daily may help. A phenothiazine compound, thiopropazate hydrochloride (Dartalan) has also been found useful in this condition. Sodium valproate (Epilim), a drug which increases the availability of GABA within the brain, has recently been shown to be of value. If confirmed, such a finding would be of considerable theoretical as well as practical importance (see Figure 4).

Where possible, reduction, or even discontinuation of neuroleptic medication is the treatment of choice for tardive dyskinesia. Elimination of symptoms may take a considerable length of time, even up to three or four years.

Autonomic effects

1 *Antiadrenergic* Most phenothiazines have a marked anti-adrenergic activity. This is particularly true for those with a piperidine side-chain such as thioridazine. These can produce severe postural hypotension leading to circulatory collapse. Raising the foot of the bed is usually sufficient to restore cerebral circulation. In extreme cases noradrenaline (*not adrenaline*) should be given by intravenous infusion.

Other cardiovascular complications of phenothiazine medication include ECG changes and frank dysrhythmias which may go on to ventricular fibrillation. These are considered to be related to a quinidine-like action of the phenothiazines, particularly thioridazine.

Of less clinical importance, but causing extreme annoyance to patients when it does occur, is failure of ejaculation. This is also more commonly a consequence of thioridazine medication than of other phenothiazines. However, this effect may be put to good use in the treatment of patients presenting with premature ejaculation (see chapter 8).

2 *Anticholinergic* As a result of the anticholinergic action of the phenothiazines, dryness of the mouth, constipation, difficulty in micturition, and blurred vision can occur.

Metabolic effects

1 *Body weight* There is often considerable weight gain noted by patients on phenothiazines, particularly chlorpromazine. The pathogensis of this is not known, but many patients report a marked increase in hunger, and this, together with the reduction in activity caused by the sedative effect of the drug, may well account for the gain in weight. This particular combination of effects is of value in the management of anorexia nervosa (see chapter 13). When it becomes troublesome a low-calorie diet should be instituted, and in some cases a non-stimulant appetite suppressant, such as fenfluramine (Ponderax) (see chapter 13) may be helpful.

2 *Endocrine* Phenothiazine drugs have been implicated as a cause of menstrual irregularity, and of lactation in non-pregnant women. Reduced libido or impotence can occur in the male.

3 *Pigmentation* Possibly as a result of the catalytic effect of ultra-violet light acting upon the melanin in the skin in the presence of phenothiazines, melanin may be deposited in the exposed skin. This leads to the purplish pigmentation in these areas which may be seen in patients receiving high doses of chlorpromazine for long periods. Melanin deposits may also be found in the cornea and in the lens of the eye. D-penicillamine in a dose of 1 g daily is said to be effective in reducing this pigmentation. In addition, thioridazine in high dosage can produce pigmentary retinopathy.

Convulsant activity

The epileptic seizure threshold is reduced by administration of phenothiazine drugs, and fits may occur even in patients without a previous epileptic history, while known epileptics show an increase in fit frequency.

Hypersensitivity reactions

1 *Cholestatic jaundice* Some patients receiving chlorpromazine develop jaundice of the cholestatic type within a few weeks of starting medication. The incidence of the complication, at one time reported to be about 1 per cent of all patients given chlorpromazine, appears to have fallen considerably in recent years. When chlorpromazine-induced jaundice does occur the drug must be stopped immediately. The jaundice then nearly always subsides spontaneously within a few weeks. If necessary, another neuroleptic drug may be given when liver function has returned to normal.

2 *Leukopenia* A fall in the total white cell count which may progress to fatal agranulocytosis occurs in a tiny minority of patients on phenothiazines (perhaps one to four in every million patients). Unfortunately, when it does happen the onset is rapid; routine monitoring of the total white cell count is therefore unlikely to pick it up in time. Any patient on phenothiazines (particularly chlorpromazine) complaining of a sore throat or fever, should have an immediate haematological investigation. If a fall in the leucocyte count is found, the drug must be stopped straight away and a full course of antibiotic treatment begun. Even with energetic treatment the mortality rate may be as high as 50 per cent. If the patient survives, extreme caution should be taken before prescribing any neuroleptic drug again.

3 *Skin reactions* Urticarial sensitivity rashes are not uncommon after neuroleptic medication. In addition, light-sensitive dermatoses may lead to an erythematous response of the exposed skin, or a more serious eczematous rash. Protecting the skin from sunlight is the only sure way of avoiding complication. Barrier creams are of limited value.

Social implications of drug treatment in schizophrenia

At about the same time as the phenothiazines were being introduced into psychiatry the social climate inside large mental hospitals was changing rapidly. The old order of impersonal custodial care gave way to the concept of more direct involvement of the patient in his own environment, leading to the development of the 'therapeutic community'. Patients were encouraged to work, at first in the hospital in well-organised industrial rehabilitation units and later in the community, either in open employment, or failing that, in sheltered workshops where the work demands could be geared to the patients' abilities. These welcome changes in attitude towards schizophrenic patients have been considerably assisted by the development of neuroleptic drugs. While many of these changes would have taken place in any case, the symptomatic relief brought about by the neuroleptic drugs has allowed the resocialisation of chronic schizophrenic patients within the community to proceed at a faster pace, and to include a greater number than would have otherwise been possible. The social and pharmacological approaches in the management of schizophrenia should be considered as complementary rather than alternatives.

Table 6   *Neuroleptic drugs*

Approved name	Proprietary name	Recommended dose (daily unless stated otherwise)	Remarks
phenothiazines 1 *aliphatic side chain*			
chlorpromazine	Largactil, Thorazine	Acutely disturbed patient: 300–900 mg Maintenance therapy: 100–500 mg	The standard phenothiazine. As effective as all other neuroleptics in the treatment of schizophrenia. But more marked tendency to produce drowsiness and risk of cholestatic jaundice and blood dyscrasias rather higher
promazine	Sparine	150–300 mg	Least effective of the phenothiazines, and more sedating. Useful for reducing disturbed behaviour in the elderly

Table 6—*Contd.*

Approved name	Proprietary name	Recommended dose (*daily unless stated otherwise*)	Remarks
trifluopro-mazine	Vesprin	20–100 mg	
acepromazine	Notensil	50–300 mg	Equal to chlorpromazine in efficacy—no advantage over other phenothiazines
propiomazine	Largon	10–40 mg	
methoxypro-mazine	Tentone		
2 *piperidine side chain*			
thioridazine	Melleril	150–600 mg	As effective as chlorpromazine with less tendency to produce extrapyramidal symptoms. More prone however to antiadrenergic effects such as hypotension and failure of ejaculation. Thioridazine can cause retinal pigmentation in prolonged dosage
mesoridazine	Serentil	100–300 mg	
piperacetazine	Quide	25–100 mg	
3 *piperazine side chain*			More extrapyramidal effects than other phenothiazines
prochlor-perazine	Stemetil	25–150 mg	The piperazine analogue of chlorpromazine to which it is clinically equivalent but produces decreased rather than increased appetite
trifluoperazine	Stelazine	10–30 mg	No advantages over other phenothiazines

Table 6—*Contd.*

Approved name	Proprietary name	Recommended dose (daily unless stated otherwise)	Remarks
thiethylperazine	Torecan	10–30 mg	Potent antiemetic
thioproperazine	Majeptil	10–40 mg	High incidence of extrapyramidal symptoms
butaperazine	Repoise	30–100 mg	No obvious advantages over other phenothiazines
perphenazine	Fentazin Trilafon	12–24 mg	
fluphenazine	Moditen Prolixin	2·5–15 mg	
fluphenazine enanthate	Moditen enanthate	12·5–25 mg every 1–3 weeks	Long-acting form given by deep intramuscular injection. Very useful in out-patient maintenance therapy of chronic schizophrenia
fluphenazine decanoate	Modecate	12·5–25 mg every 2–4 weeks	
thiopropazate	Dartalan Dartal	15–30 mg	Equal in efficacy to chlorpromazine. May relieve symptoms of persistent dyskinesia
pericyazine	Neulactil	7·5–90 mg	Said to be useful in the management of character disorders
metho-trimeprazine	Veractil	15–100 mg	No obvious advantage over the other phenothiazines
acetophenazine	Tindal	40–80 mg	
carphenazine	Proketazine	40–400 mg	

Table 6—*Contd.*

Approved name	Proprietary name	Recommended dose (daily unless stated otherwise)	Remarks
thioxanthenes			
chlorprothixene	Taractan	50–300 mg	Thioxanthene analogue of chlorpromazine. Possibly slightly inferior to chlorpromazine in acute schizophrenia
clopenthixol	Sordinol	100–400 mg	Thioxanthene analogue of perphenazine to which it may be equal in efficacy, although also said to be inferior to chlorpromazine
thiothixene	Navane	10–30 mg	Thioxanthene analogue of thioproperazine. As effective as phenothiazines but prone to cause extrapyramidal effects
flupenthixol	Fluanxol	3–12 mg	Thioxanthene analogue of fluphenazine to which it is equal in efficacy
flupenthixol decanoate	Depixol	20–40 mg every 1–3 weeks	Long-acting form of flupenthixol useful for maintenance therapy of chronic schizophrenia. Possibly less likely to cause depression than fluphenazine decanoate
indole derivatives			
oxypertine	Integrin	20–60 mg	Equal to phenothiazines in efficacy in schizophrenia. Effective in lower dose in treatment of anxiety

Table 6—*Contd.*

Approved name	Proprietary name	Recommended dose (daily unless stated otherwise)	Remarks
molindone	——	10–20 mg	Possibly slower-acting than phenothiazines in acute schizophrenia
dibenzodiazepines clozapine	Leponex	150–300 mg	Effective in schizophrenia, causes few extrapyramidal effects, but can produce marked hypotension
dibenzothiazepine metiapin	——	100–300 mg	
benzoquinolizine tetrabenazine	Nitoman	75–150 mg	Less effective than chlorpromazine in schizophrenia. May be useful in tardive dyskinesia
butyrophenones haloperidol	Serenace Haldol	1–12 mg	As effective as phenothiazines in schizophrenia, but very prone to cause extrapyramidal symptoms. Said to be particularly effective in mania. In low dosage may help in anxiety
trifluperidol (triperidol)	Triperidol	1–3 mg	Possibly among the most effective neuroleptics, having been shown to be superior to chlorpromazine, but not to trifluoperazine

Table 6—*Contd.*

Approved name	Proprietary name	Recommended dose (daily unless stated otherwise)	Remarks
benperidol (benzperidol)	Frenactil	2–6 mg	Less effective than chlorpromazine in schizophrenia. Appears to reduce sexual drive, and thus may be of some use in the treatment of sexual offenders
diphenylbutyl-piperidines			
pimozide	Orap	4–40 mg	As effective as phenothiazines in schizophrenia. Main advantage is that it only needs to be given once daily. Also effective in maintenance treatment of chronic schizophrenia
fluspirilene	Imap Redeptin	2–6 mg weekly	Long-acting compound. Administered once weekly by intramuscular injection. Used in maintenance therapy of chronic schizophrenia
penfluridol	Semap	20–50 mg weekly	Long-acting oral compound—apparently one weekly dose affords adequate maintenance therapy in chronic schizophrenia but tends to produce extrapyramidal symptoms

Suggestions for further reading

Schizophrenia—general

FISH, F., 'Clinical presentation and classification of schizophrenia', in *Contemporary Psychiatry*, ed. T. Silverstone and B. Barraclough, *British Journal of Psychiatry*, Special Publication no. 9, 1975.

HAMILTON, M., *Fish's Schizophrenia*, Wright, Bristol, 1976.

Neurochemistry of schizophrenia

ANGRIST, B., THOMPSON, H., SHOPSIN, B., and GERSHAW, S., 'Clinical studies with dopamine receptor stimulants', *Psychopharmacologia*, vol. 44, 1975, pp. 273–80.

CROW, T. J., JOHNSTONE, E. C., and MCCLELLAND, H. A.. 'The coincidence of schizophrenia and Parkinsonism: some neurochemical implications', *Psychological Medicine*, vol. 6, 1976, pp. 227–33.

DAVIS, J., 'Catecholamines and psychosis', in *Catecholamines and Behaviour*, vol. 2, ed. A. J. Friedhoff, Plenum Press, New York, 1975, pp. 135–54.

KETY, S. S., 'Biochemistry of the major psychoses', in *Comprehensive Textbook of Psychiatry*, ed. A. M. Freedman, H. I. Kaplan and B. J. Sadock, Williams & Wilkins, Baltimore, 1975.

MATTHYSE, S., 'Dopamine and the pharmacology of schizophrenia: the state of the evidence', *Journal of Psychiatric Research*, vol. 11, 1974, pp. 107–13.

POST, R. M., FINK, E., CARPENTER, W. T., and GOODWIN, F. K., 'Cerebrospinal fluid amine metabolites in acute schizophrenia', *Archives of General Psychiatry*, vol. 32, 1975, pp. 1063–9.

SMYTHIES, J. R., 'Recent progress in schizophrenia research', *Lancet*, vol. 2, 1976, pp. 136–9.

SNYDER, S. H., 'The dopamine hypothesis of schizophrenia: focus on the dopamine receptor', *American Journal of Psychiatry*, vol. 133, 1976, pp. 197–202.

Pharmacology of neuroleptic drugs

ANDÉN, N. E., BUTCHER, S. G., CORRODI, H., FUXE, F., and UNGERSTEDT, U., 'Receptor activity and turnover of dopamine and noradrenaline after neuroleptics', *European Journal of Pharmacology*, vol. 11, 1970, pp. 303–14.

ANTLEMAN, S. M., SZECHTMAN, H., CHIN, P., and FISHER, A. E., 'Inhibition of tyrosine hydroxylase but not dopamine-beta-hydroxylase facilitates the action of behaviourally ineffective doses of neuroleptics', *Journal of Pharmacy and Pharmacology*, vol. 28, 1976, pp. 66–8.

BOBON, D. P., JANSSEN, P. A. J., and BOBON, J., *The Neuroleptics*, Karger, Basle, 1970.

BUNNEY, W. E., and AGHAJANIAN, G. K., 'A comparison of the effects of chlorpromazine, 7-hydroxychlorpromazine and chlorpromazine sulf-oxide on the activity of central dopaminergic neurones', *Life Sciences*, vol. 15, 1974, p. 309.

CARLSSON, A., 'Antipsychotic drugs and catecholamine synapses', *Journal of Psychiatric Research*, vol. 11, 1974, pp. 57–64.

CROW, T. J., DEAKIN, J. F. W., and LONDON, A., 'Do anti-psychotic drugs act by dopamine receptor blockade in the nucleus accumbens ?', *British Journal of Pharmacology*, vol. 52, 1976, pp. 60–1.

CURRY, S. H., 'Chlorpromazine: concentration in plasma, excretion in urine and duration of effect', *Proceedings of the Royal Society of Medicine*, vol. 64, 1971, pp. 285–9.

MELTZER, H. Y., and FANG, V. S., 'The effect of neuroleptics on serum prolactin in schizophrenic patients', *Archives of General Psychiatry*, vol. 33, 1976, pp. 279–86.

SCHOOLER, N. R., SAKALIS, G., CHAN, T. L., GERSHON, S., GOLDBERG, S. C., and COLLINS, P., 'Chlorpromazine metabolism and clinical response in acute schizophrenia', in *Pharmacokinetics of Psychoactive Drugs*, ed. L. A. Gottschalk and S. Merlis, Spectrum, New York, 1976, pp. 199–219.

WILES, D. H., KOLAKOWSKA, T., MCNEILLY, A. S., MANDLEBROTE, B. M., and GELDER, M. G., 'Clinical significance of plasma chlorpromazine levels. 1. Plasma levels of the drug, some of its metabolites and prolactin during acute treatment', *Psychological Medicine*, vol. 6, 1976, pp. 407–15.

Drug treatment in schizophrenia

COLE, J. O., 'Phenothiazine treatment in acute schizophrenia', *Archives of General Psychiatry*, vol. 10, 1964, pp. 246–61.

DAWSON, D. A. W., 'The expectation of outcome from maintenance therapy in chronic schizophrenic patients', *British Journal of Psychiatry*, vol. 128, 1976, pp. 246–50.

FALLOON, I., WATT, D. C., and SHEPHERD, M., 'A controlled trial of Pimozide and fluphenazine decoanate', *Psychological Medicine*, vol. 8, 1978, pp. 59–70.

FOTTRELL, E., SHEIKH, M., KOTHARI, R., and SAYED, I., 'Long-stay patients with long stay drugs. A case for review: A cause for concern', *Lancet*, vol. 2, 1976, pp. 81–2.

GROVES, J. E., and MANDEL, M. R., 'The long-acting phenothiazines', *Archives of General Psychiatry*, vol. 32, 1975, pp. 893–900.

HOLLISTER, L. E., OVERALL, J. E., KIMBELL, I., and POKORNY, A., 'Specific indications for different classes of phenothiazines', *Archives of*

General Psychiatry, vol. 30, 1974, pp. 94–9.

LEFF, J. P., and WING, J. K., 'Trial of maintenance therapy in schizophrenia', *British Medical Journal*, vol. 3, 1971, pp. 559–604.

PINDER, R. M., BROGDEN, R. N., SAWYER, P. R., SPEIGHT, T. M., SPENCER, R., and AVERY, G. S., 'Pimozide: a review of its pharmacological properties and therapeutic uses in psychiatry', *Drugs*, vol. 12, 1976, pp. 1–40.

SINGH, M., and KAY, S. R., 'A longitudinal therapeutic comparison between two prototypic neuroleptics (haloperidol and chlorpromazine) in matched groups of schizophrenics', *Psychopharmacologia*, vol. 43, 1975, pp. 115–23.

SWAZEY, J. P., *Chlorpromazine in Psychiatry*, MIT Press, Cambridge, Mass., 1974.

Unwanted effects of neuroleptic drugs

CRANE, G. E., 'Persistent dyskinesia', *British Journal of Psychiatry*, vol. 122, 1973, pp. 395–405.

HOLLISTER, L. E., 'Adverse reactions to phenothiazines', *Journal of the American Medical Association*, vol. 189, 1964, pp. 311–13.

KLETT, C. J., and CAFFEY, E., 'Evaluating the long term need for antiparkinsonian drugs by chronic schizophrenics', *Archives of General Psychiatry*, vol. 25, 1972, pp. 374–9.

LITVAK, R., and KAELBLING, R., 'Agranulocytosis, leukopenia and psychotropic drugs', *Archives of General Psychiatry*, vol. 24, 1971, pp. 265–7.

MINDHAM, R. H. S., 'Assessment of drug induced extrapyramidal reactions and of drugs given for their control', *British Journal of Clinical Pharmacology*, vol. 3, 1976, pp. 395–400.

PEELE, R., and VON LOETZEN, I. S., 'Phenothiazine deaths: a critical review', *American Journal of Psychiatry*, vol. 130, 1973, pp. 306–9.

7   Affective disorders

And men should know that from the brain comes joys, delights, laughter and jests, and sorrows, griefs, despondency and lamentations.

Hippocrates

Introduction

The affective disorders are those conditions in which there is alteration of mood to such a degree as to cause serious distress or disruption of normal life. The mood may be abnormally elevated as in mania, or lowered as in depression. Depression may either be a symptom of reaction to adverse circumstances, or an illness in its own right. The tendency to confuse the symptom with the illness has in the past led to certain conceptual difficulties. We all get depressed (symptom) from time to time when things go wrong; this is a perfectly natural reaction. Some people react rather more frequently and sharply than others, but the quality of their *depressive reaction* does not differ from our own. A few people, however, (1–2 per cent of the population) develop a much more serious condition—a true *depressive illness* which, as often as not, comes completely out of the blue with no obvious precipitating cause. A number of labels have been given to this illness: 'melancholia', 'psychotic depression', 'the depressive phase of a manic-depressive psychosis', 'endogenous depression', and, when it comes on later in life, 'involutional melancholia'. Essentially, however, they are all similar in their manifestation and the basic treatment approach is the same for each. Only when states of depression alternate with episodes of mania should the term manic-depressive psychosis be used. Some authors refer to the depressive phase of this particular variant as 'bipolar' depression, reserving 'unipolar' depression for those cases in which mania has not previously appeared.

Psychopathology

Depressive illness

This can be described as a persistent alteration of mood, exceeding customary sadness, which characteristically comes on 'out of the blue' with no obvious environmental precipitant. It is usually accompanied by one or more of the following symptoms: self-deprecation and a morbid sense (or delusional ideas) of guilt; sleep disturbance (typically early morning awakening); retardation of thought or action; agitated behaviour; suicidal ideas or attempts at suicide; an inability to concentrate and lack of interest in the surroundings; profound anorexia with consequent weight loss. It does not change with alteration in environmental circumstance and requires treatment with drugs or electroconvulsive therapy (ECT).

Depressive reaction

This, on the other hand, can clearly be seen to arise as the direct result of some unfortunate circumstance in the patient's life. Typically the patient blames others for his misfortune rather than himself. (In contrast, the patient with depressive illness is usually riddled with self-blame.) In a depressive reaction there are no delusional ideas, severe retardation is uncommon and successful suicide occurs far less frequently. The sleep disturbance is characteristically a difficulty in getting off to sleep rather than early morning waking. Although anorexia may occur in some patients, others turn to food for comfort and thus gain, rather than lose, weight. Finally, depressive reactions readily respond to environmental changes, and if the precipitating circumstances can be alleviated further treatment often proves unnecessary.

Mania

Mania occurs less frequently than depression. It is characterised by over-activity both day and night, loss of social inhibitions and lack of judgment leading to self-assertiveness, over-generosity and recklessness. In addition, the manic patient has a sense of well-being and talks non-stop in a continuous stream of jokes, puns and personal remarks, which very soon become extremely wearisome to the listener. While some cases abort spontaneously, most require medical intervention.

Biochemical basis of affective disorders

Both depressive illness and mania are associated with biochemical changes in the brain and other parts of the body which are of importance in pathogenesis and in the further development of the disorder. These changes involve particularly the brain amines, the electrolytes sodium and potassium, and certain hormones, particularly thyroid and adrenocorticosteroid hormones.

Monoamines

Following the largely unexpected observations that imipramine, a drug originally synthesised as a neuroleptic, had pronounced anti-depressant activity, and that iproniazid, a drug used in the treatment of tuberculosis, had euphoriant properties (see chapter 1), a determined effort was made to understand how these drugs acted in the brain, in the hope of discovering the neurochemical basis of the affective disorders. It was a case of empirical treatments in search of rational explanations.

Imipramine was found to inhibit the neuronal reuptake of noradrenaline (NA) and 5-hydroxytryptamine (5 HT) by presynaptic neurones in the CNS (see chapter 3). Iproniazid was shown to inhibit the enzyme monoamine oxidase within the neurone; this enzyme is responsible for metabolising all three neurotransmitter monoamines. Subsequently this and other compounds with similar inhibitory activity on monoamine oxidase came to be known as monoamine oxidase inhibitors (MAOI).

At about the same time, reserpine, a compound which had been introduced in the early 1950s for the treatment of hypertension, was noted to cause symptoms resembling a severe depressive illness in a number of patients. Examination of its action in the CNS revealed that reserpine depleted the brain stores of the three monoamine neurotransmitters, NA, dopamine (DA) and 5HT. Thus, a drug which depleted the brain of monoamines caused depression, while drugs which increased the available monoamine neurotransmitters at the receptor, either by blocking their reuptake (the dibenzazepines) or by preventing their metabolism (the MAOI), elevated mood. These observations gave rise to what has come to be known as the monoamine theory of depression, which may be stated as follows:

Depression is due to an absolute or relative *decrease* in mono-amines, or of receptor sensitivity, at certain receptor sites in the brain, whereas mania is due to an absolute or relative *excess* of monoamines, or an increase in receptor sensitivity, at these sites.

Stated in such general terms this theory still has some validity. Unfortunately it offers no clues as to which receptor sites or which monoamines are involved. In any case depression is unlikely to be a unitary condition. Genetically, bipolar depression can be distinguished from unipolar, and this genetic distinction is paralleled by biochemical differences between the two types of depression. For example, levodopa, the precursor of dopamine, can produce symptoms of mania in patients with bipolar depression but not in those with unipolar depressive illness. This would suggest that DA is involved in bipolar, but not in unipolar depression. In other words bipolar depression may be associated with a decrease in DA activity, and mania might be associated with an increase. The finding that pimozide, a specific dopamine receptor blocking compound, is effective in mania is consistent with such a view. Unipolar depression on the other hand may be due to a reduction in the activity of either a NA system, or a 5HT system, or both.

Some depressed patients have a lowered level of 5HIAA (the metabolite of 5HT) in their CSF which would imply a relative lack of 5HT in the CNS. Van Praag has reported that these patients do well following treatment with drugs such as chlorimipramine which preferentially block the neuronal reuptake of 5HT, or with 5-hydroxytryptophan (5HTP) a precursor of 5HT, and do even better with a combination of the two. In a proportion of depressed patients the CSF 5HIAA remains low after recovery. Kety has suggested that the lowered level of brain 5HT 'permits' affective change to occur, but in itself is not sufficient to bring it about. The fact that some manic patients also have 'lowered' 5HIAA in the CSF, suggests that the lowered 5HIAA is not merely a reflection of the underlying mood state. Consistent with the view that 5HT is involved in depressive illness was the finding that the brain of depressed patients who had committed suicide had a lowered concentration of 5HT in the brain stem; however, some doubt has recently been cast on these observations, as it has been shown that post mortem changes can bring about a similar reduction in brain 5HT.

Noradrenaline has been imputed to be involved in the pathogenesis of depressive illness by a number of authorities. This view is based on the finding that the urinary concentration of the metabolites of NA, 3 methoxy, -4-hydroxy—phenylglycol (MHPG) and vanilylmandelic acid (VMA) were reduced in depressed patients. Subsequent investigations suggested that the reduction in these metabolites of NA was secondary to the generalised reduction in overall motor activity which occurs in retarded depressed patients. In any case there is no firm evidence that even the CSF MHPG level is a true reflection of NA activity in the brain; it may be more closely related to spinal cord activity. Yet, in spite of these doubts concerning the role of NA in depression it should be stated that the drugs which appear to act most rapidly in depressive illness, drugs such as protriptyline and maprotiline, are believed to act largely if not entirely on the NA system. Furthermore amphetamine, which can alleviate depressive symptoms in a number of patients, albeit for a short time, acts almost exclusively on the catecholamines NA and DA. It may well be that unipolar depressive illness can arise as a consequence of a number of biochemical abnormalities; in some patients it may well be due to changes in the 5HT system, in others the NA system may be affected, while in yet others altogether different neurotransmitter systems might play a part. The possible involvement of cholinergic neurones should not be overlooked. Blockade of central choline esterase with physostigmine can produce lethargy and dysphoria in normal subjects; similar treatment in patients with mania ameliorates their symptoms.

Electrolytes

In 1932 Gjessing showed that changes in water and electrolyte balance accompanied cyclic affective disorders in some patients. Since that time numerous studies have been carried out with conflicting results, because, although marked changes were demonstrated, no consistent pattern was associated with particular mental states in different patients.

The distribution of electrolytes in the cells and extracellular fluid has a profound influence on neuronal activity with the resting potential dependent on the ratio of the concentration of potassium inside and outside the cell, and the action potential dependent on the ratio of the concentrations of intracellular to extracellular sodium. Calcium and magnesium ions also have marked effects on nerve cell membranes and on release of neurotransmitters. It would not be surprising, therefore, if changes in concentration and distribution of electrolytes throughout the body, and particularly in the brain, were associated with changes in neuronal function and were reflected in disorders of behaviour and mood.

Evidence to support the belief that electrolytes do play a role in the pathogenesis of the affective disorders comes from the finding that lithium salts appear to have a prophylactic value in reducing the incidence and severity of recurrent mania and depression. It is not unlikely that these effects depend at least partly on its marked action on sodium transport across cell membranes, which change the distribution of sodium and chloride between the intra- and extracellular fluid spaces.

Endocrine function

While profound psychological changes may accompany all endocrine disorders, thyroid and adrenal cortical dysfunction in particular are associated with changes in mood. It is possible that thyroid hormone influences central nervous activity through changes in adenylcyclase, an enzyme identical to, or closely related to, the adrenergic receptor. Thyroid hormone stimulates adenylcyclase, which in turn leads to an increase in cyclic AMP. It is reasonable to suppose that changes in concentration of adenylcyclase and cyclic AMP in the brain may underlie some if not all of the psychological changes associated with a deficiency or excess of thyroid hormone.

A relationship between depression and adrenal cortical activity is suggested first by the clinical observation that states of profound depression may be produced by administration of high doses of corticotrophin or cortisol. Second, patients with severe endogenous depression may themselves frequently have raised plasma cortisol levels throughout the 24 hours, with a loss of normal diurnal variation. This is probably due, in turn, to an increased pituitary corticotrophin production which may depend on disordered hypothalamic control of anterior pituitary function. Looking at it the other way round, patients with Cushing's syndrome, whose primary abnormality is a raised level of circulating corticosteroids, frequently become profoundly depressed; this depression is improved dramatically when their endocrine state is returned to normal.

Amine metabolism, electrolyte balance and thyroid and adrenal cortical function are all interrelated, and it is not yet possible to say whether changes in one or more of them are responsible for, or the result of, an affective disorder. If the monoamine hypothesis, or a variant of it, is correct then it might be envisaged that alterations in electrolyte distribution would modify neuronal excitability and transmitter release and uptake. Changes in neuronal activity in the hypothalamus might influence pituitary and adrenal cortical function to change the rate of cortisol production which in turn would produce further changes in electrolyte balance. Changes in thyroid function could modify monoamine activity, as has already been said, by altering brain levels of adenylcyclase and cyclic AMP. However, the way in which these biochemical events are linked to changes in mood and affect remains unknown.

Pharmacology

Drugs for depression

It follows from the monoamine theory of depression that successful treatment of depression should be associated with an increase in central monoamine activity. This could theoretically be achieved by four different pharmacological mechanisms (see chapter 2), (1) monoamine reuptake inhibition, (2) monoamine oxidase inhibition, (3) monoamine release and (4) phosphodiesterase inhibition.

1 *Monoamine reuptake inhibiting drugs (MARI)* This category of drugs includes those compounds which are commonly known as the 'tricyclic antidepressants'. They have many pharmacological properties including anticholinergic, anti-5HT, antihistamine, hypothermic and antiemetic actions. Their antidepressant activity, however, is probably due to their ability to block the neuronal uptake of catecholamines and 5HT thus increasing the effective concentrations of these monoamines at central receptor sites, even though the brain amine content is not increased. It is probable that these compounds have both an acute action and a longer term chronic effect. After a single dose they inhibit the uptake of noradrenaline and 5HT in the animal brain and may also prevent deamination by monoamine oxidase in the mitochondria. They also inhibit the pressor response to tyramine in man, and the uptake of dopamine into human platelets after administration of single doses. After administration of MARI to experimental animals for several days the uptake of monoamines is still reduced, and the levels of their metabolites are also reduced (as after acute administration). In contrast to the acute experiments, however, their rate of disappearance is *not* reduced, suggesting increased turnover. Furthermore, chronic administration of MARI as well as of

monoamine oxidase inhibitors, and of ECT to experimental animals results in a reduction in activity of the noradrenergic cyclic AMP generating system in the limbic forebrain. It may be that it is these delayed changes in monoamine turnover and in receptor activity which underly the therapeutic activity of MARI in man, which does not usually come on until several days after administration.

Many MARI also potentiate the peripheral pressor effect of noradrenaline and adrenaline, as well as affecting their central actions. This peripheral action assumes particular importance in patients given injections of local anaesthetic preparations which contain these catecholamines, and other directly-acting sympathomimetic pressor amines, as vaso-constrictor agents. Another important peripheral interaction of MARI is with antihypertensive drugs such as guanethidine, bethanidine and debrisoquine which block noradrenaline release after being taken up into the noradrenergic neurone. The uptake of these drugs, like that of noradrenaline, is blocked by MARI, and so their antihypertensive effect is reduced or abolished.

Many MARI possess potent anticholinergic activity, which may be related to their clinical effect, particularly if, as has been suggested, there is a disturbance of central cholinergic activity in depressive illness. Such anticholinergic activity may also underly the cardiotoxic effect of some of these drugs.

Imipramine is the parent compound of the group, and is metabolised within the body to its demethyl derivative desipramine. Many related compounds have now been introduced, and it is claimed, largely on the basis of animal studies, that some possess selectivity of action in blocking the uptake of one monoamine rather than another; secondary amines (e.g. desipramine, protriptyline) appear to be more potent than tertiary amines (e.g. imipramine, amitriptyline) in blocking NA uptake whereas the tertiary amines are generally more potent in blocking 5HT uptake. Nomifensine is somewhat unusual in blocking DA as well as NA reuptake. This generalisation, however, is complicated by the problem of extent and routes of metabolism of the parent compound in man. Extensive metabolism to compounds with different uptake-blocking profiles may occur in man through routes different from those in animals. This consideration obviously throws considerable doubt on conclusions relating to clinical action in patients reached from *in vitro* studies in animal tissue with the parent compound alone. And in man there is considerable genetic variability with regard to metabolism, and hence to the plasma level reached after a given dose (see chapter 3). Whether or not such variation in plasma levels is related to clinical efficacy is uncertain; some authors have described a linear relationship between plasma level and clinical response, others have described an inverted 'U' shaped relationship in which higher doses appear to be less effective, and finally yet other authors have found no relationship at all between plasma levels and therapeutic effect.

The term 'tricyclic' which was applied to these drugs was always inappropriate, because other groups of centrally acting compounds such as the phenothiazines also possess a tricyclic nucleus (page 95). However, the term has become even more inappropriate with the introduction of tetracyclic antidepressive compounds such as maprotiline and mianserin, and bicyclic compounds such as viloxazine, the majority of which share with the tricyclic compounds the basic pharmacological property of central monoamine reuptake inhibition. There is a wide spectrum of peripheral pharmacological activity among these drugs, ranging from a relative lack of anticholinergic and peripheral noradrenaline reuptake blocking effects with drugs such as mianserin and viloxazine, to the profound anticholinergic and peripheral reuptake blocking properties of amitriptyline.

Other drugs may interfere with the metabolism of the MARI antidepressants and thus influence their clinical effects. For example, phenothiazines, such as chlorpromazine (see chapter 6) may block their hydroxylation, thereby increasing their plasma levels and potentiating their therapeutic activity and their side effects.

Although the principal type of monoamine reuptake is into monoaminergic neurones (Uptake $_1$) a second form of uptake also occurs by diffusion into other, non-neuronal tissues (Uptake $_2$). There is some evidence to suggest that corticosteroids may inhibit the uptake$_2$ process, and if this occurs in the central nervous system, then it may account, at least in part, for their euphoriant and anti-depressant activity in debilitated and terminally-ill patients.

2   *Monoamine oxidase inhibitors* (*MAOI*)   Inhibition of the intracellular enzyme monoamine oxidase (MAO) leads to an increase of the monoamines noradrenaline, dopamine and 5HT in the

brain. Any antidepressant effect MAO inhibitors may have would fit in well with the monoamine hypothesis. Many other drugs inhibit MAO to a limited extent, including cocaine and amphetamine, but their pharmacological actions do not appear to depend on this effect. The compounds in which antidepressant effects probably depend on MAO inhibition fall into two chemical groups: (i) those which are hydrazine derivatives, particularly toxic to the liver (isocarboxazid, nialamide and phenelzine) and (ii) those related to amphetamine, the most important being tranylcypromine which appears to have intrinsic sympathomimetic activity of its own. Some of this latter group of drugs, particularly tranylcypromine are also potent inhibitors of noradrenaline uptake. It is, therefore, uncertain to what extent an increased level of noradrenaline at the receptor site produced by tranylcypromine is due to inhibition of metabolic degradation of noradrenaline on the one hand and to inhibition of uptake on the other.

Monoamine oxidase is not a single entity but a group of more specific enzymes, each of which is concerned with an individual monoamine. Most of the monoamine oxidase inhibitors in general use inhibit the whole family of enzymes and thus lead to an increase in all the monoamines. However, certain MAOI, such as clorgyline, have been claimed, on the basis of animal experiments, to inhibit preferentially the enzyme responsible for one monoamine rather than another; but clinical pharmacological studies in man have failed to demonstrate this selectivity of action.

MAO is important in the handling of many drugs and foodstuffs within the body. For this reason, drugs which inhibit the enzyme complex may have important interactions with it.

(a) *Sympathomimetic amines* After MAO inhibition, the indirectly acting amines may evoke enhanced effects both peripherally and centrally. Many easily available proprietary remedies for upper respiratory tract infections contain such amines, and thus patients taking MAO inhibitors must be cautious in their use.

(b) *Certain foodstuffs* Foods which contain pressor amines such as dopa and tyramine may produce hypertensive reactions in patients receiving MAO inhibitors. These include broad beans, which contain dopa, and certain cheeses containing large quantities of tyramine. Under normal circumstances most tyramine ingested by mouth is metabolised immediately by MAO in the intestinal mucosa and liver. Following MAO inhibition, the absorption of tyramine is increased markedly and it rapidly enters the circulation to cause prolonged release of noradrenaline and thus evoke pressor effects. Some wines, yeast products and animal livers also contain significant amounts of tyramine.

(c) *Central nervous depressant drugs* The central effects of pethidine and other narcotic compounds are prolonged in patients receiving MAOI, and excitation, rigidity, coma, changes in blood pressure, hyperpyrexia and shock may occur. This interaction can be prevented in animals by drugs such as p-chlorophenylalanine which prevent the intracerebral accumulation of 5HT but not by compounds which reduce noradrenaline synthesis. It appears, therefore, that an increase in brain 5HT is necessary for this interaction to occur.

(d) *Antihypertensive drugs* Some of the antihypertensive drugs, including guanethidine and bethanidine, may release noradrenaline from peripheral sympathetic nerve endings when administered in high concentration, for example, intravenously. In the absence of MAO activity, these compounds may release increased amounts of noradrenaline on to receptor sites and produce hyperexcitation and hypertension.

(e) *Monoamine reuptake inhibiting drugs* Antidepressant drugs, such as imipramine as described above, inhibit uptake of noradrenaline and possibly 5HT into central nerve terminals, thus increasing their activity at receptor sites. It would be expected on theoretical grounds, therefore, that MAO inhibitors might potentiate their effects, and this has been demonstrated in animal experiments. There have also been reports of serious reactions in patients treated with a combination of these two groups of compounds.

3 *Monoamine releasing drugs* The indirectly acting sympathomimetic amines such as amphetamine and phenmetrazine, together with some other drugs such as methylphenidate and pemoline, probably produce central stimulation by release of dopamine and noradrenaline from, and to some extent by blockade of uptake into NA and DA neurones. In addition, amphetamine may have a direct central dopamine receptor stimulant action. Their central stimulant effect is seen in an increase of alertness and in motor and psychological activity, together with a decrease in fatigue and varying degrees of insomnia. These effects have led to the widespread abuse of amphetamine and phenmetrazine, and these two drugs are now subject to legal restrictions in many

countries. Chronic use of this group of drugs in large doses may ultimately lead to alarming psychotic symptoms with paranoid features.

These drugs cannot be considered to be as therapeutically useful antidepressive drugs as are the MARI and MAOI, because their central effects lead to anxiety, restlessness and agitation rather than normality of mood. This may be because they enhance central catecholamine activity without increasing activity of 5HT.

4 *Phosphodiesterase inhibitors* The enzyme phosphodiesterase is responsible for inactivating cyclic AMP which is thought to be intimately involved with mediating noradrenergic and dopaminergic receptor activity (chapter 2). Drugs which inhibit phosphodiesterase would, therefore, be expected to increase cyclic AMP activity and produce effects similar to central catecholamine activity. The methylxanthines such as caffeine, theophylline and theobromine are phosphodiesterase inhibitors, and have central stimulant properties reducing fatigue and augmenting the capacity for physical excretion. Excessive administration produces insomnia, restlessness, anxiety, headache and tremor, and dependence may develop. As with the monoamine releasing drugs, they cannot be considered as therapeutically useful antidepressive drugs.

ECT Electroconvulsive therapy (ECT) still remains the most effective form of antidepressant treatment for severe cases. If the monoamine theory is true, then it would be expected that this form of treatment should also influence central monoamine activity. Its effect on cerebral amines in man are not known, but animal studies have shown a reduction in brain levels of noradrenaline in ECT-treated animals compared with untreated controls, suggesting that this procedure may increase neuronal discharge of noradrenaline in the brain. Furthermore, normetadrenaline levels were higher than in the controls, and as this metabolite is the result of COMT activity this would indicate an increased extraneuronal breakdown after release onto receptors.

Drugs for mania

Two types of drugs are of value in the treatment of mania, the neuroleptic compounds and lithium.

1 *Neuroleptic drugs* The pharmacology of these drugs is considered in chapter 6. Suffice it to say here that their effectiveness in

mania may be explained in terms of the monoamine theory by their ability to block post synaptic catecholaminergic receptors, particularly dopamine.

2 *Lithium* Lithium is the lightest of the alkali earth elements, coming below sodium, potassium, rubidium and caesium in terms of atomic weight. In the body it imperfectly substitutes for sodium and potassium ions and consequently it can have profound effects on a great number of metabolic processes. While substitution by lithium for potassium and sodium may underly its more severe toxic effects such as convulsions and coma, this is not thought to be the basis for its psychotropic activity. Toxic symptoms begin to occur when the serum concentration exceeds 1·5 mM/L, so every effort, including regular serum estimations, must be made to ensure that this upper level of 1·5 mM/L is not exceeded. Especial care should be taken whenever there is a possibility of fluid or electrolyte imbalance as in the case of persistent vomiting or diarrhoea.

Within the central nervous system lithium reduces the neurotransmitter-induced activation of adenylate cyclase at certain post synaptic receptors. Normally the neurotransmitters noradrenaline and dopamine activate adenylate cyclase, and this in turn catalyses the formation of cyclic adenosine monophosphate (AMP) from adenosine triphosphate (ATP). AMP is frequently referred to as the 'second messenger' for in many cells it mediates the changes within those cells produced by circulating hormones ('first messengers'). In the CNS the catecholamine neurotransmitters are acting similarly to hormones in the periphery, that is they are behaving as first messengers, while cyclic AMP acts as the second messenger. The reduction by lithium of the formation of cyclic AMP within cells acted upon by catecholamine neurotransmitters would be in keeping in terms of the monoamine hypothesis, with the clinical observation that lithium is effective in mania (see section on treatment of mania). It would not, however, explain any antidepressant activity that lithium may possess, nor does it fully explain its well-documented prophylactic properties (see section on prophylaxis of affective disorders). The effects of lithium on adenylate cyclase is not limited to the CNS. Other organs, notably the thyroid gland and the kidney can also be affected. In the thyroid the release of thyroid hormone from the gland induced by thyroid stimulating hormone (TSH) is mediated by cyclic AMP, and can be inhibited by lithium. The subsequent impairment of thyroxine release can, in time, lead to the development of a frank hypothyroid syndrome. In the kidney the action of antidiuretic hormone (ADH) is mediated via cyclic AMP. Lithium, by reducing adenylate cyclase activity, interferes with the antidiurectic effect of ADH, and, as a result, there is an increased flow of dilute urine, or polyuria; a condition referred to as nephrogenic diabetes insipidus.

Although a number of cyclic AMP systems in other tissues have been shown in experimental animals to be affected by lithium, the clinical implications, if any, of such findings are as yet unknown.

Treatment

Depression

When presented with a patient who is unhappy, perhaps weeping, obviously distressed, and who gives a history of inability to cope, a sense of hopelessness perhaps with suicidal ideas, profound anorexia and marked insomnia, it is necessary to determine first of all the likely underlying cause for these symptoms, and secondly to assess their severity. Treatment varies considerably according to the type of condition present (i.e. whether it is a true depressive illness or a depressive reaction to distressing circumstances), and to its severity. If the patient is so desperate that there is a real risk of a suicide attempt, or if he is so incapacitated by his symptoms as to be unable to care for himself adequately, hospitalisation is likely to be necessary, followed by treatment with electroconvulsive therapy (ECT). Where the patient is neither suicidal nor incapacitated, it will usually be possible to treat him with the appropriate medication as an out-patient. Although in many cases it is not possible to distinguish categorically between a depressive illness and a depressive reaction, an attempt to do so should be made, as the treatment is different for each. Depressive illness usually responds well to one of the MARI antidepressant drugs, whereas depressive reactions often respond more rapidly to an anxiolytic sedative rather than an antidepressant. Where the distinction between depressive illness and reaction cannot be made with any confidence, treatment should proceed as for depressive illness. In cases of so-called 'atypical' depression, particularly if there is a lengthy history, with failure to respond to MARI antidepressants, monoamine oxidase inhibitors may prove effective.

Depressive illness (endogenous depression)

1   *Monoamine reuptake inhibiting drugs (MARI)*   The so-called tricyclic antidepressant drugs, together with certain newer, non-tricyclic antidepressant compounds are believed to act by blocking the reuptake of monoamines from the synaptic cleft, hence the term monoamine reuptake blocking drugs (MARI), (see pages 126–8). There is a large number of such drugs available (see Table 7). They are all of similar efficacy, some 60–70 per cent of patients improve on them, compared to 30–40 per cent who improve on placebo and 70–80 per cent who improve on ECT. Patients who respond best are those suffering from a clear cut depressive illness of moderate severity, with a history of less than six months' duration. Although the majority of MARI take some ten to fourteen days to become fully effective, at least two, protriptyline (Concordin, Vivactil) and maprotiline (Ludiomil) appear to act more quickly.

Among the factors which influence the metabolism and plasma levels of these drugs, and hence their efficacy, are genetic predisposition, other drugs being administered at the same time (particularly barbiturate and phenothiazine compounds), and pH (acidification of the urine leading to faster excretion).

In general all the members of this group of drugs have similar side-effects, the commonest being due to the pronounced anticholinergic properties they possess. These effects include dryness of the mouth, excessive sweating, postural hypotension which may lead to falling, difficulty in visual accommodation, constipation and urine retention. More dangerous are the cardiovascular effects. It is not uncommon to find a prolonged QT interval in the electrocardiogram in patients being treated with tricyclic antidepressants. This can proceed to a frank dysrhythmia or ventricular tachycardia, which in cases of overdose occasionally progresses to fatal ventricular fibrillation. In the elderly, congestive cardiac failure is not uncommon. In addition to these autonomic and cardiac effects, the tricyclics are epileptogenic and may precipitate epileptic seizures in those who are otherwise predisposed. In view of all these possible side-effects, MARI drugs should be used most cautiously in patients with glaucoma, prostatism, chronic heart disease and epilepsy. Certain of the newer MARI drugs such as maprotiline, mianserin (Bolvidon, Norval) and viloxazine (Vivalan) would seem less likely to cause anticholinergic side effects than their predecessors. Mianserin is also less likely to produce untoward cardiovascular effects. Viloxazine produces less drowsiness than other MARI but it does have a greater tendency to cause nausea. Maprotiline has been reported to precipitate epilepsy rather more frequently than other antidepressants.

The choice of drug to use in any particular case depends on a number of factors. Efficacy is similar for all the marketed products (see Table 7 for effective dose regimes for individual drugs). Where they differ is in speed of action, sedative effects and side-effects. The two most rapidly acting MARI drugs, protriptyline and maprotiline, have obvious advantages when, as in most cases, speed of action is important; however protriptyline has pronounced anticholinergic activity and it must be used with caution in patients in whom such effects may be of serious consequence, for example in patients with a history of glaucoma or of urinary retention. Maprotiline on the other hand appears to be well tolerated and might be considered as suitable for most cases of depression other than those with a history of epilepsy.

Some patients exhibit overwhelming anxiety and restless agitation during the course of a depressive illness. In such cases it is obviously an advantage to have a compound which, in addition to its antidepressant activity, has a pronounced sedative effect. Amitriptyline (Tryptizol, Elavil), together with its oxepin and thiapin analogues, doxepin (Sinequan) and dothiepin (Prothiaden), do have this combination of actions and are thus particularly useful in the anxious, depressed patient. Nomifensine (Merital) is also said to possess pronounced anxiolytic properties. While there are also a variety of mixtures combining an antidepressant with an anxiolytic sedative (amitriptyline with chlordiazepoxide [Limbitrol]; amitriptyline with perphenazine [Triptafen]; nortriptyline with perphenazine [Motival]; imipramine with promazine), we would not recommend their use. If the addition of an anxiolytic sedative is thought necessary then one of the benzodiazepine group of drugs (see chapter 8) can be prescribed as required, allowing a greater flexibility of dosage.

The other MARI compounds listed in Table 7 would not appear to have any distinct advantages over those already discussed. It is better to become familiar with the dosage and effects of some two or three compounds and stick to them; for instance imipramine (or perhaps maprotiline if its early clinical promise is maintained) as the standard antidepressant, amitriptyline or one of its analogues (see above) for the patient with endogenous depression who is also anxious, dothiepin when autonomic side-effects need to be reduced to a minimum, and mianserin when the risk of cardiac complications is high.

Once a patient has responded well to ECT or to a tricyclic antidepressant he should be maintained on a lower dose of MARI drug for some six months after recovery in order to minimise the risk of relapse. Some patients with previous recurrent depressive illness have been maintained symptom free for at least two years on continuous treatment with MARI drugs.

2 *Monoamine oxidase inhibitors (MAOI)* From the evidence provided from well-controlled clinical trials it would appear that MAOI are not as effective as the tricyclic antidepressants in depressive illness. In addition they have the serious disadvantages of producing hypertensive reactions with certain foods, interacting with drugs like pethidine and causing liver damage. Occasionally, however, they can produce remissions in patients where all else has failed. The available drugs in this group are listed in Table 7. Particular caution should be maintained when changing from a MAOI to a tricyclic antidepressant or vice versa. It is safest to allow a two week drug-free interval between the two.

L-tryptophan, the amino-acid precursor of 5HT, in a dose of 5–9 g per day, has been reported to increase the efficacy of MAOI in depression, possibly by increasing the availability of 5HT at the synaptic junction.

3 *Neuroleptic drugs* Certain neuroleptic compounds have been used in depressive illness. While some studies have revealed that chlorpromazine (Largactil, Thorazine) and flupenthixol (Fluanxol) are useful in the treatment of depressive illness, most authorities would recommend starting treatment with a tricyclic drug rather than a neuroleptic.

4 *Lithium* Lithium was originally introduced as a treatment for mania but some workers have claimed that it is also effective in certain cases of depressive illness (particularly 'bipolar' depression). In general, however, lithium is not as effective as the MARI compounds in depressive illness.

Depressive reactions (reactive depression, neurotic depression)
As we have already indicated, depressive reactions, in contrast to depressive illness, respond more readily to anxiolytic sedatives

than to antidepressants, although those antidepressant drugs with a pronounced sedative action, such as amitriptyline and doxepin, or nomifensine with its additional anxiolytic effect, may be effective. They are especially useful when it is uncertain which type of depression is present.

The choice of the appropriate anxiolytic sedative to use in this condition lies largely among the benzodiazepine groups of drugs (see chapter 8). In addition counselling and supportive psychotherapy should form an integral part of the treatment programme.

Mania

1 *Neuroleptic drugs* The manic patient, with his non-stop activity, constant pressure of talk, bellicose self-confidence and inability to focus on any activity for more than a moment, will nearly always require urgent treatment, preferably in hospital. The neuroleptic drugs (see chapter 6), particularly the phenothiazine compound chlorpromazine (Largactil, Thorazine), the butyrophenone, haloperidol (Serenace, Haldol) and the diphenylbutylpiperidine compound, pimozide (Orap) have proved to be very effective in the treatment of mania.

Initially, if the patient is unwilling to take oral medication, intramuscular administration of some 250–500 mg chlorpromazine or 10–30 mg haloperidol will be required. This may need to be repeated until the patient becomes sufficiently cooperative to take the drug orally. It is usually a matter of trial and error to determine the dose which is adequate to control the symptoms without being too sedating. For chlorpromazine it is likely to lie between 75 and 200 mg three times daily, for haloperidol to be between 5 mg and 30 mg twice daily and for pimozide 4–20 mg daily. Such high doses of neuroleptics may produce marked parkinsonian effects which can be alleviated by antiparkinsonian drugs such as benzhexol (Artane) 2–4 mg three times daily, or orphenadrine (Disipal) 50–100 mg three times daily (see chapter 6).

Medication should be continued for several weeks after the patient has returned to normal, when it can be cautiously reduced. However, should any of the signs of mania reappear, treatment will then need to be maintained at a higher dose for another period of several weeks.

2 *Lithium* Although lithium was introduced as an effective treatment for mania as early as 1949, by Cade in Australia, it was

used very little until the late 1960s. It would appear from well-controlled trials that lithium carbonate has a definite therapeutic effect in mania, but this effect usually takes about a week to appear. As there is such a relatively long delay in onset of action, lithium is not particularly useful as the sole initial treatment in mania because of the need for a drug with a much more rapid action (see above). It can, however, be given at the same time as a neuroleptic, and the neuroleptic can then be gradually tailed off as the lithium takes effect.

When administering lithium carbonate, either as the standard tablet (Camcolit) or as the longer acting preparations (Priadel, Phasal) it is essential to ensure that the plasma levels remain below 1·5 milli-moles per litre. Lithium carbonate would appear to be at least as reliable in obtaining the required plasma levels as the longer acting formulations. Above this level toxic effects appear, and above 2 mM/L these toxic effects can prove extremely dangerous (see below). On the other hand, in order to ensure that an effective dose is being given, it is advisable to maintain the plasma level of lithium above 0·6 mM/L. Thus the safe but effective range of plasma lithium levels is 0·6–1·5 mM/L. It is necessary to monitor plasma levels frequently (at least weekly) for the first few weeks of treatment.

Once the appropriate dose has been established to maintain adequate plasma levels then blood level estimations need only be repeated monthly or even less frequently unless the patient develops an intercurrent illness.

Early signs of toxicity include a fine tremor of the hands and a sensation of nausea or abdominal discomfort. If the plasma level of lithium rises further it can lead to drowsiness, vomiting and diarrhoea; at this point lithium should be stopped immediately and the blood level measured as a matter or urgency. If this is not done the clinical state may deteriorate further with coma and death ensuing. With severe lithium poisoning haemodialysis may be necessary. Under no circumstances should lithium be administered to a patient with a history of serious renal or cardiac disease, and it should only be given with great circumspection to a patient with hypothyroidism, as lithium interferes with thyroid metabolism, and can produce frank myxoedema.

Other unwanted effects of lithium treatment include production of a reversible nephrogenic diabetes insipidus which appears to be due to inhibition of vasopressin sensitive adenylate cyclase.

Patients with this condition complain of disturbed sleep and may need to pass urine four or five times nightly. Treatment consists of reduction of the dose of lithium or administration of a thiazide diuretic which paradoxically has an antidiuretic effect in this condition.

Sodium loss results in lithium retention and the risk of intoxication. This underlies the potentially dangerous interaction of lithium with diuretics, particularly the more potent agents such as frusemide.

Prophylaxis of affective disorders

Many patients who have a depressive illness or an attack of mania give a history of previous episodes of either mania or depression. These periods of illness tend to become more frequent with time, eventually occurring once or twice a year. It would obviously be of considerable benefit to such patients if these attacks of affective disorder could be prevented. Schou and his colleagues in Denmark have presented convincing evidence that continuous administration of lithium carbonate (maintaining a plasma level of between 0·6 and 1·5 mM/L) significantly reduces the relapse rate. These Danish findings have now been confirmed by other investigators. Therefore patients with recurrent attacks of depressive illness (*not* depressive reactions or neurotic depression) and mania should be given a trial of lithium prophylaxis. The dosage required to maintain adequate blood levels will be similar to that used in the treatment of mania (see above), i.e. 0·6 to 1·5 g per day. Any signs of toxicity (see above) should be an indication for checking the serum level, and if necessary stopping the drug for a few days. As before, no patients with serious cardiac or renal disease should be treated with lithium and care must be taken in cases where there is any suggestion of hypothyroidism. With these provisos, suitable patients may be safely and successfully maintained on lithium medication for years.

Although lithium significantly reduces the recurrence rate of manic depressive disorders, and reduces the severity of those attacks which do occur, it is by no means always successful. In one study some 45 per cent of patients with rapidly cycling manic depressive illness relapsed while on lithium, the majority relapsing within the first six months of treatment, in spite of adequate plasma levels. Nevertheless the success rate in preventing relapse was much greater with lithium than without. Some authorities have suggested that it is the level of lithium inside the erythrocyte, rather than the level in the plasma which is important, and that monitoring the intra-erythocyte lithium concentration might reduce the relapse rate still further.

While lithium is generally agreed to be the most effective available prophylactic agent for bipolar depression (manic-depressive illness), there is less certainty about its value in preventing recurrences of unipolar depression. Here a case can be made out for long-term maintenance with a MARI drug, although the relative efficacy of MARI as compared to lithium maintenance in recurrent unipolar depressive illness has yet to be fully determined.

Table 7 *Antidepressant drugs*

Approved name	Proprietary name	Recommended dose (daily unless stated otherwise)	Remarks
monoamine reuptake inhibiting drugs			
imipramine	Tofranil	75–200 mg	The 'standard' tricyclic compound against which others are compared. Autonomic and cardiac effects may be pronounced at higher dosage. Takes 10–14 days to act
desipramine	Pertofran Norpramine	75–200 mg	The demethylated metabolite of imipramine; no advantages over imipramine
trimipramine	Surmontil	50–100 mg (as single dose before retiring)	Methylated derivative of imipramine; no obvious advantages over other tricyclics

Table 7—*Contd.*

Approved name	Proprietary name	Recommended dose (*daily unless stated otherwise*)	Remarks
clomipramine (chlorimipramine)	Anafranil	50–150 mg (can be given as infusion)	Chloro-derivative of imipramine; no obvious advantages over imipramine. Can be given by intravenous infusion. Said to be useful in obsessional and phobic disorders
amitriptyline	Tryptizol Elavil	75–200 mg	Effective antidepressant with sedative properties, particularly useful in depressive illness accompanied by anxiety. Takes 10–14 days to act fully
	Lentizol	50–100 mg sustained release tablets at night	
butriptyline	Evadyne	50–150 mg	No proven advantage over amitriptyline
nortriptyline	Aventyl	75–200 mg	Demethylated derivative of amitriptyline; no obvious advantage over amitriptyline
protriptyline	Concordin Triptil Vivactil	15–60 mg	Unsaturated analogue of nortriptyline; the most rapidly acting of the tricyclics. Effective within 5–10 days
doxepin	Sinequan	75–150 mg	Oxepin derivative of amitriptyline. Pronounced anxiolytic effect. Antidepressant activity equal to imipramine and amitriptyline

Table 7—*Contd.*

Approved name	Proprietary name	Recommended dose (*daily unless stated otherwise*)	Remarks
dothiepin	Prothiaden	75–150 mg	Thiapin derivative of amitriptyline. As effective as amitriptyline with fewer autonomic side-effects
iprindole	Prondol	45–90 mg	An indole central ring with imipramine side-chain. As effective as imipramine and amitriptyline with fewer autonomic effects. May cause liver damage
opipramol	Insidon Ensidon	100–150 mg	Imipramine nucleus with piperazine side-chain. No advantage over imipramine
dibenzepin	Noveril	240–480 mg	Structure resembles imipramine with side-chain in different position. Clinically equivalent to imipramine
maprotiline	Ludiomil	50–150 mg	Rapidly acting anti-depressant with relatively low incidence of anti-cholinergic side effects. May precipitate epileptic attack in predisposed individual.
mianserin	Bolvidon Norval	20–60 mg	Equal efficacy to amitriptyline with less anticholinergic side effects and less danger of cardiotoxicity

Table 7—*Contd.*

Approved name	Proprietary name	Recommended dose (*daily unless stated otherwise*)	Remarks
nomifensine	Merital	50–150 mg	Equal in efficacy to imipramine with greater anxiolytic activity
viloxazine	Vivaian	100–300 mg	Equal in efficacy to imipramine with less drowsiness and anticholinergic side effects. Prone to cause nausea
Monoamine oxidase inhibitors			Little convincing evidence of efficacy in depressive illness, although certain patients respond well.
1 *hydrazines*			All MAOI can cause severe hypertensive
phenelzine	Nardil	30–60 mg	reaction with tyramine-
isocarboxazid	Marplan	20–40 mg	containing foods (e.g.
nialamide	Niamid	50–150 mg	cheese), sympatho-
mebanazine	Actomol	5–30 mg	mimetic amines and
iproniazid	Marsilid	50–75 mg	tricyclic antidepressants. Also potentiate action of
2 *non-hydrazines*			pethidine and alcohol. May cause liver damage. Of some value in
tranyl-cypromine	Parnate	20–40 mg	management of phobic disorders. Maybe genetically determined slow acetylators respond best to phenelzine due to reduced rate of metabolism of the drug.

Suggestions for further reading

Neurochemistry of affective disorders

ASBERG, M., THOREN, P., TRASKMAN, L., BERTILSSON, L., and RINGBERGER, v., '"Serotonin depression"—a biochemical subgroup within the affective disorders', *Science* vol. 191, 1976, pp. 478–80.

ASHCROFT, G. W., 'Modified amine hypothesis for the aetiology of affective illness', *Lancet*, vol. 2, 1972, pp. 573–7.

BALDESSARANI, R. J., 'The basis for amine hypothesis in affective disorders', *Archives of General Psychiatry*, vol. 32, 1975, pp. 1087–93.

BUNNEY, W. E., GERSHON, E., MURPHY, D., and GOODWIN, F. H., 'Psychological and pharmacological studies of manic depressive illness', *Journal of Psychiatric Research*, vol. 9, 1972, pp. 207–26.

KETY, S. S., 'Biochemistry of the major psychoses', in *Comprehensive Textbook of Psychiatry*, ed. A. M. Freedman, H. I. Kaplan and B. J. Sadock, Williams & Wilkins, Baltimore, 1975.

LANCET Editorial, 'Adrenergic-cholinergic imbalance in affective disorders', *Lancet*, vol. 2 1976, p. 1342.

MAAS, J. W., 'Biogenic amines and depression', *Archives of General Psychiatry*, vol. 32, 1975, pp. 1357–61.

MENDELS, J., STERN, S., and FRAZER, A., 'Biochemistry of depression', *Diseases of the Nervous System*, vol. 37 (Number 3, Section 2), 1976, pp. 3–9.

MENDELS, J., and FRAZER, A., 'Reduced serotonergic activity in mania', *British Journal of Psychiatry*, vol. 126, 1975, pp. 241–8.

MURPHY, D. L., and REDMOND, D. E., 'The catecholamines: possible role in affect, mood and emotional behaviour in man', *Catecholamines and Behaviour*, vol. 2, ed. A. J. Friedhoff, Plenum Press, New York, 1975, pp. 73–117.

SCHILDKRAUT, J. J., 'Neuropharmacology of the affective disorders', *Annual Review of Pharmacology*, vol. 15, 1973, pp. 427–54.

SHAW, D. M., RILEY, G., TIDMARSH, S., and BLAZER, R., 'Unipolar affective illness', *Lancet*, vol. 1, 1976, pp. 363–8.

Pharmacology of antidepressant drugs

ALEXANDERSON, B., and SJOQVIST, F., 'Individual differences in the pharmacokinetics of non-methylated tricyclic antidepressants: role of genetic and environmental factors and clinical importance', *Annuals of the New York Academy of Science*, vol. 179, 1971, pp. 1739–51.

GHOSE, K., COPPEN, A., and TURNER, P., 'Autonomic actions and interactions of mianserin hydrochloride and amitriptyline in patients with depressive illness', *Psychopharmacology*, vol. 49, 1976, pp. 201–4.

GHOSE, K. GIFFORD, L. A., TURNER, P., and LEIGHTON, M., 'Studies of the interaction of desmethylimipramine with tyramine in man, after a single oral dose, and its correlation with plasma concentrations', *British Journal of Clinical Pharmacology*, vol. 3, 1976, pp. 334–7.

JOHNSON, A. M., LOEW, D. M., and VIGOURET, J. M., 'Stimulant properties of bromocriptine on central dopamine receptors in comparison to apomorphine, amphetamine and l-dopa', *British Journal of Pharmacology*, vol. 56, 1976, pp. 59–68.

NYBACK, H. V., WALTERS, J. R., AGHAJANIAN, G. K., and ROTH, R. H., 'Tricyclic antidepressants: effects on the firing rate of brain noradrenergic neurons', *European Journal of Pharmacology*, vol. 32, 1975, pp. 302–12.

SALT, P. J.. 'Inhibition of noradrenaline uptake in the isolated rat heart by steroids, clonidine and methoxylated phenylethylamines', *European Journal of Pharmacology*, vol. 20, 1972, pp. 329–40.

TRENCHARD, A., TURNER, P., PARE, C. M. B., and HILLS, M., 'The effects of protriptyline and clomipramine *in vitro* on the uptake of 5-hydroxytryptamine and dopamine in human platelet-rich plasma', *Psychopharmacologia*, vol. 43, 1975, pp. 89–93.

Treatment of depression

BAN, T. A., 'Pharmacotherapy of depression—a critical review', *Psychosomatics*, vol. 16, 1975, pp. 17–20.

BERGER, F. M., 'Depression and antidepressant drugs', *Clinical Pharmacology and Therapeutics*, vol. 18, 1975, pp. 241–8.

KILOH, L. G., BALL, J. R. B., and GARSIDE, R. F., Prognostic factors in treatment of depressive states with imipramine', *British Medical Journal*, vol. 1, 1962, p. 1225.

MEDICAL RESEARCH COUNCIL, 'Clinical trial of the treatment of depressive illness', *British Medical Journal*, vol. 1, 1965, pp. 881–6.

MINDHAM, R. H. S., HOWLAND, C., and SHEPHERD, M., 'An evaluation of continuation therapy with tricyclic antidepressants in depressive illness', *Psychological Medicine*, vol. 3, 1973, pp. 5–17.

PAYKEL, E. S., 'Depressive typologies and response to amitriptyline', *British Journal of Psychiatry*, vol. 119, 1971, pp. 555–64.

PAYKEL, E. S., and TANNER, J., 'Life events, depressive relapse and maintenance treatment', *Psychological Medicine*, vol. 6, 1976, pp. 481–5.

Plasma levels of antidepressant drugs and response to treatment

ASBERG, M., CRONHOLM, B., SJOQVIST, F., and TUCK, D., 'Relationship between plasma level and therapeutic effect of nortriptyline', *British Medical Journal*, vol. 3, 1971, pp. 331–4.

BRAITHWAITE, R. A., GOULDING, R., THEANO, G., BAILEY, J., and COPPEN, A., 'Plasma concentrations of amitriptyline and clinical response', *Lancet*, vol. 2, 1972, pp. 1297–300.

PEREL, J. M., SHOSTAK, M., GANN, E., KANTOR, S. J., and GLASSMAN, A. H., 'Pharmacodynamics of imipramine and clinical outcome in depressed patients', in *Pharmacokinetics of Psychoactive Drugs*, ed. L. A. Gottschalk and S. Merlis, Spectrum, New York, 1976, pp. 229–41.

ZIEGLER, V. E., CO, B. T., TAYLOR, J. R., CLAYTON, P. J., and BIGGS, J. T., 'Amitriptyline levels and therapeutic response', *Clinical Pharmacology and Therapeutics*, vol. 19, 1976, pp. 795–801.

Newer antidepressant drugs

A. Maprotiline

POTTER, P. A., 'A clinical double-blind comparison of maprotiline and amitriptyline in depression', *Current Medical Research and Opinion*, vol. 3, 1976, pp. 634–41.

REIGER, W., RICKLES, K., NORSTAD, N., and JOHNSON, J., 'Maprotiline and imipramine in depressed in-patients', *Journal of International Medical Research*, vol. 3, 1975, pp. 413–16.

SILVERSTONE, J. T., CARNE, H. J., DELL, A., FRANKLIN, C. J., SWIRSKY, S. N., and FORREST, W. A., 'A comparison of maprotiline and amitriptyline in the treatment of depression in general practice', *Practitioner*, vol. 218, 1977, pp. 279–82.

B. Mianserin

COPPEN, A., GUPTA, R. MONTGOMERY, S., GHOSE, K., BAILEY, J., BURNS, B., and DE RIDDER, J. J., 'Mianserin hydrochloride: a novel antidepressant', *British Journal of Psychiatry*, vol. 129, 1976, pp. 342–5.

MURPHY, J. E., 'A comparative clinical trial of mianserin and imipramine in the treatment of depression in general practice', *Journal of International Medical Research*, vol. 3, 1975, pp. 251–60.

WHEATLEY, D., 'Controlled clinical trial of a new antidepressant (Mianserin) of novel chemical formulation', *Current Therapy Research*, vol. 18, 1975, pp. 849–54.

C. Nomifensine

FORREST, A., HEWETT, A., and NICHOLSON, P., 'A controlled randomised group comparison of nomifensine and imipramine in depressive illness', *British Journal of Clinical Pharmacology*, vol. 4, supplement 2, 1977, pp. 215s–220s.

D. Viloxazine

BAYLISS, P. F. C., DEWSBURY, A. R., DONALD, J. F., HARCUP, J. W., MAYER, M., MILLION, R., MOLLA, A. L., MURPHY, J. E., PLANT, B., and SHAOUL, E., 'A double-blind controlled trial of viloxazine hydrochloride and imipramine hydrochloride in the treatment of depression in general practice', *Journal of International Medical Research*, vol. 4, 1974, pp. 260–4.

MAGNUS, R. V., 'A placebo controlled trial of viloxazine with and without tranquillisers in depressive illness', *Journal of International Medical Research*, vol. 3, 1975, pp. 207–13.

TSEGOS, I. K., and EKDANI, M. Y., 'A double-blind controlled study of viloxazine and imipramine in depression', *Current Medical Research and Opinion*, vol. 2, 1974, pp. 455–60.

Toxic effects of antidepressant drugs

BURROWS, G. D., VOHRA, J., HUNT, D., SLOMAN, J. G., SCOGGINS, B. A., and DAVIES, B., 'Cardiac effects of different tricyclic antidepressant drugs' *British Journal of Psychiatry*, vol. 129, 1976, pp. 335–41.

JEFFERSON, J. W., 'A review of the cardiovascular effects and toxicity of tricyclic antidepressants', *Psychosomatic Medicine*, vol. 37, 1975, pp. 160–79.

Drug treatment of mania

COOKSON, J., and SILVERSTONE, T., '5-hydroxytryptamine and dopamine pathways in mania: a pilot study of fenfluramine and pimozide', *British Journal of Clinical Pharmacology*, vol. 3, 1976, pp. 942–43.

Lithium

CRAMMER, J. L., ROSSER, R. M., and CRANE, G., 'Blood levels and management of lithium treatment', *British Medical Journal*, vol. 3, 1974, pp. 650–4.

DAVIS, J. M., 'Maintenance therapy in psychiatry: II affective disorders', *American Journal of Psychiatry*, vol. 133, 1976, pp. 1–13.

DUNNER, D. L., FLEISS, J. L., and FIEVE, R. R., 'Lithium carbonate prophylaxis failure', *British Journal of Psychiatry*, vol. 129, 1976, pp. 40–4.

DUNNER, D. L., STALLONE, F., and FIEVE, R. R., 'Lithium and affective disorders; a double-blind study of prophylaxis of depression in bipolar illness', *Archives of General Psychiatry*, vol. 33, 1976, pp. 117–20.

GLEN, A. I. M., 'Lithium: its indications, use and clinical implications', in *Advanced Medicine—Topics in Therapeutics*, vol. 2, ed. P. Turner, Pitman, London, 1976, p. 190.

GERSHON, S., and SHOPSIN, B., *Lithium, its Role in Psychiatric Research and Treatment*. Plenum Press, New York, 1973.

JOHNSON, F. N., *Lithium Research and Therapy*, Academic Press, London, 1975.

LADER, M., 'Lithium', *Prescribers Journal*, vol. 16, 1976, pp. 63–8.

PRIEN, R. F., CAFFEY, E. M., and KLETT, C. J., 'Comparison of lithium carbonate and chlorpromazine in the treatment of mania', *Archives of General Psychiatry*, vol. 28, 1973, pp. 337-41.

QUITKIN, F., RIFKIN, A., and KLEIN, D. F., 'Prophylaxis of affective disorders', *Archives of General Psychiatry*, vol. 33, 1976, pp. 337-41.

SCHOU, M., AMDISEN, A., and BAASTRUP, P. C., 'The practical management of lithium treatment', *British Journal of Hospital, Medicine* vol. 6, 1971, pp. 53-60.

TYRER, S., HULLIN, R. P., BIRCH, N. J., and GOODWIN, J. C., 'Absorption of lithium following administration of slow-release and conventional preparations', *Psychological Medicine*, vol. 6, 1976, pp. 51-8.

Anxiety

8

Anxiety is an inevitable by-product of the process by which a person learns to become a member of society. . . . The fact that the human being can experience fear permits this learning to take place. In the process anxiety arises.

Levitt

Psychophysiology of anxiety

Anxiety and fear play a vital role in all human societies. To feel anxious in the face of a threatening stimulus is both normal and appropriate; it is only when the anxiety becomes so severe as to be incapacitating, or arises without reasonable cause, that clinical intervention is indicated. Unfortunately this occurs all too frequently. In a large epidemiological survey in the London area it was found that 14 per cent of the population at risk consulted the doctor at least once during the course of a year for symptoms which were a reflection of underlying anxiety. A Scandinavian study revealed that one-third of the adult population had overt symptoms of anxiety, nervousness or tension; 5 per cent had symptoms severe enough to warrant the diagnosis of an anxiety state.

The subjective awareness of anxiety and fear is associated with general 'arousal' of the central nervous system plus peripheral autonomic discharge. Stimuli which are seen as threatening produce activation of the reticular activating system (RAS) in the brain stem, probably via corticofugal pathways passing down from the cerebral cortex to the reticular formation, the cortex classifying the particular stimuli as being threatening or not. It is likely that the cerebral cortex and the RAS together constitute a feedback-control system maintaining an optimal arousal level. Through this system when cortical activity is great the RAS activity is inhibited, thereby preventing too great an arousal level. Should this inhibition of the RAS break down then the cortical activity may continue unchecked, leading to a state of incapacitating anxiety.

In addition other areas of the brain are clearly involved in the pathogenesis of anxiety, particularly the structures grouped in the limbic system, including the amygdala and the hippocampus, together with areas in the hypothalamus. Stimulation of the posterior hypothalamus in laboratory animals leads to behaviour suggestive of a panic reaction; stimulation of the same area in humans is reported as being most unpleasant. It is believed that the hypothalamic centres, which probably regulate the autonomic discharge seen in anxiety, are themselves under the control of the hippocampus and amygdala; on the one hand the amygdala increases, and on the other the hippocampus and septal region inhibits the hypothalamic response to threatening stimuli.

It has been found that stimulation of the centro-medial hypothalamus in a normally placid cat will generate aggressive behaviour which can be considerably modified by simultaneous stimulation of the amygdala. Furthermore, such electrical stimulation of the amygdala produces a rapid rise in 17-hydroxycorticosteroids presumably by increasing ACTH production via the hypothalamic pituitary axis.

Additional experimental evidence for the view that these regions of the brain are important in the production of anxiety comes from studies using implanted electrodes. When electrodes are placed in certain areas of the brain of a rat (e.g. the septal region and the lateral hypothalamus), and the animal can turn on the current by pressing a lever with its foot (self-stimulation), it is repeatedly found that the rat will continuously stimulate itself in this way for hours at a time, ignoring food and water. If an animal has been trained to expect a shock on hearing a click it will normally cower in a corner of its cage when the click sounds. If however it is able to self-stimulate its septal area it will ignore the sound of the click and even when the electric shock is applied to its feet it will not show any sign of a fear reaction; it just keeps on self-stimulating.

The hippocampal–amygdala system is in turn regulated by the cerebral cortex which, as we have seen, is modulated by the RAS through a feedback loop.

Histochemical studies have shown that the neurones of the lower brain stem, where the RAS is situated, contain noradrenaline (NA) and dopamine (DA). These particular neurones have widespread synaptic connections with the limbic system and it has been postulated that NA may act as the transmitter in the system underlying anxiety responses, particularly as the NA levels in NA cells rise during the performance of a conditioned avoidance response. In addition to the NA cells in the lower brain stem there are others projecting to the lateral hypothalamus and the hippocampus which synthesise 5-hydroxytryptamine (5HT). It could be that these two cell types themselves act reciprocally, the NA cell system increasing the anxiety response and the 5HT cell system reducing it. In keeping with this hypothesis is the finding that members of the benzodiazepine group of drugs (see below) which are effective in the treatment of anxiety, can increase brain 5HT levels, and promote the release of gamma-aminobutyric acid (GABA), a neurotransmitter which probably inhibits noradrenergic activity.

Whatever the central mechanism involved, the subjective experience of anxiety is usually accompanied by widespread sympathetic discharge together with a steep rise in circulating catecholamines. The particular autonomic changes which have been most studied are those occurring in the cardiovascular system and those in the palmar sweat glands.

Increased anxiety has long been known to be associated with a quickening of the heart. Measurements of peripheral blood flow, using venous occlusion plethysmography, have demonstrated that when an individual is anxious his forearm blood flow also increases. These autonomic responses can reinforce the central awareness of anxiety and thus compound the severity of the symptoms; such cardiovascular concomitants frequently cause the patient to seek medical advice.

The palmar sweat glands, which have little thermoregulatory function, are innervated by the sympathetic nervous system but, unlike the rest of this system, are cholinergic rather than adrenergic. Thus drugs blocking adrenergic responses (i.e. the beta-adrenergic blockers—see below) do not affect increased palmar sweating although they can effectively reduce psychogenic tachycardia. The level of palmar sweating determines the electrical resistance of the palmar skin. When sweating is marked, resistance is low, and vice versa. This phenomenon is the basis of the so-called psychogalvanic response (see chapter 4) which has proved to be a most useful physiological variable with which to compare states of psychological arousal.

The autonomic accompaniments of anxiety are so pervasive that at one time it was thought that they, rather than any central phenomena, actually caused the anxiety. This view was shown to be erroneous by Cannon and it came to be accepted that the experience of anxiety was entirely dependent on the central state, with little reference to what was occurring peripherally.

This was too great a swing of the pendulum, as Schachter showed. In a series of ingenious experiments he revealed that it is the *interaction* between peripheral autonomic events and the central nervous system which determine the specific emotional response observed in a particular situation. When normal subjects received injections of adrenaline and were told what to expect (i.e. tachy-cardia, etc.) they did not experience marked emotions even in the face of provocation, whereas those subjects who were not informed what to expect in the way of physiological changes reacted much more vigorously to amusing situations as well as to threatening ones. Schachter concluded that the autonomic events increase central arousal, but the way the individual behaves when aroused is determined by what is happening around him. If he is in a threatening situation he becomes angry or fearful, whereas if he is in an amusing situation he becomes happy. In summary, the direction of the emotion experienced is determined by the nature of the situation and the personality of the individual, while the amplitude of the emotional response is modified by the degree of autonomic discharge.

Pharmacology of anxiolytic-sedative drugs

Drugs used in the treatment of anxiety states may be divided broadly into two groups, namely those which act primarily on the central nervous system and those which block peripheral autonomic receptors.

Centrally acting drugs

These are known as anxiolytic sedatives (sometimes referred to as minor tranquillisers). There is as yet no purely anxiolytic compound, all have some sedative properties.

1   *Benzodiazepine drugs*   These drugs have been introduced into clinical medicine relatively recently, but have already established themselves as a major advance in the treatment of anxiety states, and their use has grown enormously in the past decade (see chapter

5). When given to animals in small doses they appear to act primarily on subcortical structures such as the amygdala and hippocampus of the limbic system, without affecting the cerebral cortex. It has been suggested, on the basis of animal experiments, that they act by increasing the level of available 5HT in these centres. Evidence has recently emerged that benzodiazepine compounds promote the release of GABA from GABA neurones. As GABA acts as an inhibitory neurotransmitter on catecholamine pathways, it may well be that the anxiolytic activity of the benzodiazepines is due to the release of GABA at the locus coeruleus; this would inhibit the dorsal NA tract, a major ascending NA pathway.

Clinically, the benzodiazepine drugs have an anxiolytic action in doses which do not produce sedation, although higher doses may cause drowsiness and lethargy. Physical as well as psychological dependence to these drugs has been described and convulsions have occurred when they have been withdrawn following prottracted administration in high doses.

Overdosage with these agents, accidentally or for suicidal purposes, produces drowsiness, sleep, inco-ordination, muscle weakness, ataxia and dysarthria. In a large series of cases of chlordiazepoxide intoxication in which the dose ingested ranged from 60 to 100 mg the patients were at no time completely unrousable. Although relatively safe when taken alone, benzodiazepines may potentiate the central depressant effects of alcohol and barbiturate drugs and such combinations can be dangerous.

There are several benzodiazepine drugs available for the treatment of anxiety. These include: chlordiazepoxide (Librium); clorazepate (Tranxene); diazepam (Valium); lorazepam (Ativan); medazepam (Nobrium); oxazepam (Serenid).

Other members of this group of compounds, nitrazepam (Mogadon) and flurazepam (Dalmane) are used as hypnotics (see chapter 11).

The metabolism of the various members of the benzodiazepine group of anxiolytic sedatives is interconnected—see Figure 6.

All appear to be rapidly absorbed after oral administration but their half-lives vary, with consequent variation in length of action. The duration of action assumes great importance when considering subjective 'hangover' symptoms, or objective psychomotor effects. For example, a compound with a longer half-life may, when taken at night as a hypnotic cause psychomotor impairment the following

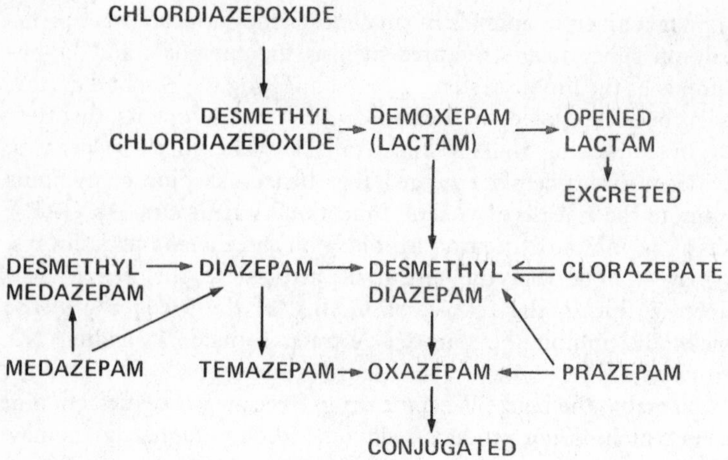

Figure 6 *The metabolic pathways of the benzodiazepines* (from M. H. Lader, in *Topics in Therapeutics*, vol. 2, ed. P. Turner, Pitman, London, 1976)

morning; this has obvious implications for car driving or handling complex machinery (see chapter 5).

2 *Barbiturate drugs* Although the most important use of the barbiturates is as hypnotics to induce sleep they are effective anxiolytic sedatives in small doses. Phenobarbitone and amylobarbitone are the most commonly used barbiturates for this purpose. While their mode of action is not clearly understood, they are known to produce widespread depression of neuronal activity throughout the brain, particularly in synapses of the reticular activating system in the brain stem. At the molecular level, the barbiturate drugs probably act by depressing formation of high energy phosphate which is essential for normal brain activity.

The ratio between the dose of a barbiturate drug, such as phenobarbitone, necessary to relieve symptoms and signs of anxiety and that which produces other evidence of central nervous depression is small. For this reason it is difficult to obtain a satisfactory anxiolytic effect without some reduction of alertness and vigilance. In some cases this may lead to marked impairment of consciousness and sleep. As the dose is increased central nervous depression becomes still more marked with the involvement of respiratory and vasomotor centres.

Apart from the dangers of overdosage, there are two other important disadvantages which barbiturates possess:

(i) a tendency to produce drug dependence
(ii) induction of liver microsomal enzymes.

Therapeutic doses of barbiturate drugs are sufficient to stimulate the activity of liver microsomal enzyme systems concerned with their own metabolism and with that of other drugs. This stimulating effect, or induction, is associated with increased liver weight, increased production of microsomal protein, and changes in the smooth membrane of the endoplasmic reticulum. Among the drugs whose half-lives are known to be reduced by treatment with barbiturate drugs are: (i) coumarin anticoagulants, leading to a reduction in their hypoprothrombinaemic effects (ii) phenytoin, reducing its anticonvulsant effect (iii) griseofulvin, the antifungal agent, (iv) coricosteroids and (v) oral contraceptives.

The most important of these interactions is with the coumarin drugs. It is not uncommon for a patient admitted to hospital following a myocardial infarction to be treated with a coumarin anticoagulant drug and also with a barbiturate such as phenobarbitone to relieve anxiety and mental distress. The latter drug, by liver enzyme induction, increases the rate of hydroxylation of the coumarin drug so reducing its anticoagulant effect, which leads in turn to an increase in the dose required to obtain the desired prolongation of prothrombin time. When the barbiturate drug is withdrawn, often when the patient leaves hospital, the microsomal enzyme activity returns to normal over a period of two or three weeks. Unless the dose of the anticoagulant drug is reduced during this period, a dangerous increase in prothrombin time may occur as its rate of metabolism returns to normal, producing a potentially dangerous haemorrhagic tendency.

Whenever a barbiturate drug is prescribed, particularly on a long-term basis, its possible interaction with other substances should be considered. Little is known of the significance or extent of enzyme induction in man, but its importance is probably much greater than has been realised.

3 *Propanediols* Meprobamate, like mephenesin from which it is derived, is a skeletal muscle-relaxing compound in experimental animals, but in addition has tranquillising properties in man. It appears that its principal mechanism of action as an anxiolytic

agent is to block activity between the cerebral cortex and sub-cortical structures, thus interfering with centrally mediated autonomic responses. In doses of about 400 mg little if any sedation occurs, but 800 mg or more has marked hypnotic properties in many patients. Several controlled trials have shown that meprobamate is superior to barbiturates as a hypnotic agent, probably because of its relative lack of hang-over effects.

Habituation occurs to meprobamate, and abstinence symptoms and epileptiform convulsions on withdrawal of the drug have been reported. Overdosage produces pronounced central nervous depression with somnolence and hypotonia, and finally coma.

Although meprobamate is widely prescribed in musculoskeletal disorders it is unlikely to be effective in reducing muscle spasm except where the spasm is due to an underlying anxiety state.

4 *Diphenylamines* The two drugs in this group, hydroxyzine and benactyzine, have now largely been superseded.

5 *Neuroleptics* ('major tranquillisers') (see chapter 6)

(i) *Chlorpromazine* (Largactil, Thorazine) This drug is not as effective in the treatment of anxiety as amylobarbitone.

(ii) *Trifluoperazine* (Stelazine) Several well-controlled studies have indicated that trifluoperazine is of some use in anxiety as well as in schizophrenia, but it would seem to possess no advantages over the benzodiazepines in this situation.

(iii) *Haloperidol* (Serenace) This drug has recently been promoted for use in anxiety. Again no particular advantage over the standard compound is apparent.

(iv) *Oxypertine* (Integrin) In contrast to the other neuroleptics this drug may have a definite place in the management of anxiety. In one study, 10 mg three times daily was found to be more effective than diazepam 5 mg three times daily, with less psychomotor disturbance; other trials however have failed to reveal any such superiority of oxypertine over diazepam.

(v) *Pimozide* (Orap) This is a member of the longer acting diphenylbutylpiperidine group of compounds. Pimozide only needs to be given once daily in a dose of 2–4 mg. Preliminary trials indicate that when given in this way it is virtually equal in efficacy to chlordiazepoxide.

6   *Other compounds: benzoctamine* (Tacitin). A molecule with an unusual steric structure, it possesses both anxiolytic and muscle relaxant properties. Its place in the management of anxiety is uncertain as yet.

A wide variety of other centrally acting drugs have at one time or another been tried in the treatment of anxiety symptoms. While many have been shown under double-blind conditions to be more effective than placebo, few, if any, are clearly better than the benzodiazepines (see Table 8).

The sedative action of alcohol should not be forgotten in transient or mild anxiety states, particularly in elderly patients. Insomnia, restlessness and nervousness may often be allayed by the judicious use of an alcoholic beverage.

Peripherally acting drugs

Many of the manifestations of anxiety already described are probably due to an increased release of adrenaline and noradrenaline from the adrenal medulla and sympathetic nerves, and changes in urinary excretion of these amines and their metabolites have been demonstrated in patients suffering from anxiety. For this reason adrenergic blockade with drugs, such as propranolol, is effective in reducing or abolishing anxiety symptoms, particularly those which are predominantly autonomic in nature like palpitations and tremor. Relatively small doses of propranolol such as 10 or 20 mg six- or eight-hourly may be used together with small doses of a benzodiazepine drug. It must be remembered that, in some patients, bronchial asthma is a manifestation of anxiety; when this happens propranolol and other beta blockers are contra-indicated.

Drug treatment of anxiety

Mild to moderate anxiety symptoms

When a patient presents with either the psychological symptoms of anxiety (excessive worrying, inability to concentrate, difficulty in getting off to sleep) or its somatic accompaniments (palpitations, tension headaches, sweaty palms), the first step is to establish whether or not there is a reasonable cause for these symptoms to arise at that particular time. If so, it may be possible for the situation to be adjusted in such a way that the anxiety-provoking circumstances no longer apply.

Recognition of the underlying cause may, therefore, be itself of considerable therapeutic benefit. If, however, as is so often the case, the causative factors cannot be defined or modified, or there are no adequate grounds for the patient's symptoms, symptomatic relief with drugs together with psychological support is the next step. Before starting drug treatment it should be determined whether or not the patient's symptoms are but an acute episode in a normally non-anxious individual, or whether they reflect a long-standing predisposition to the development of frequent, perhaps even continuous, anxiety. In the former situation it is likely that remission will occur without any definitive therapeutic intervention. 40–50 per cent of such cases have been shown to remit spontaneously, although anxiolytic sedative drugs may increase this remission rate still further. In contrast, patients with chronic anxiety symptoms will more frequently require drug treatment, often for considerable periods of time, and at a dosage greater than patients with acute anxiety.

Of the available compounds the benzodiazepines are the drugs of choice. The benzodiazepine compounds are as effective as the barbiturates and are certainly safer. However they are not without pronounced sedative effects and can produce marked ataxia. Whether one member of this group of drugs possesses any distinct advantages over the others is open to question. When comparisons have been made between them it has usually been on the basis of fixed dosages, so that the finding that diazepam 5 mg three times daily is more effective than chlordiazepoxide 10 mg three times daily does not necessarily imply that an increased dose of chlordiazepoxide would not be better still. Probably the benzodiazepine of first choice should be diazepam, with a dose ranging from 2 mg twice a day in a patient with mild symptoms, or in an elderly patient, to 20 mg three or four times a day in a patient with incapacitating anxiety (see below). Of the others, oxazepam (10 to 15 mg two to four times a day) would appear to possess some theoretical advantage over diazepam which is itself metabolised to oxazepam in the body. Fine adjustment of dosage can often be left to the individual patient who is usually in the best position to judge the optimum dose for his symptoms. It is illogical and unnecessary to prescribe more than one benezodiazepine compound at a time.

When there is a pronounced cardiovascular element in the symptomatology, with one of the patient's main complaints being tachycardia, it may be helpful to prescribe a beta-adrenergic blocking compound in addition to the anxiolytic sedative. Propranolol 10 to 20 mg three or four times a day has been shown to be effective; other compounds in this group like oxprenolol and sotalol may also prove of value.

Severe anxiety state

When a patient presents with symptoms of anxiety so severe that he is incapable of functioning at all effectively either at work or at home it is necessary, whatever the cause and whatever the underlying personality, to reduce the level of central arousal as rapidly as possible. In extreme cases parenteral administration of an anxiolytic sedative may be initially required; either amylobarbitone sodium 300 mg intramuscularly or diazepam 10 mg intravenously. Subsequent large doses of oral medication should be prescribed for the first few days: a benzodiazepine such as diazepam 15 to 20 mg four times daily; or oxazepam 15–30 mg three times daily. Additional sedation at night is usually needed (see chapter 11).

When the patient has been adequately sedated (and such a regime may well require hospitalisation) the dosage of drugs can be reduced gradually to a level where little or no daytime drowsiness is produced.

Some patients who present with an anxiety attack severe enough to warrant such measures may eventually be able to do without any medication, but most will require long-term administration of an anxiolytic sedative in the dosages recommended for mild to moderate anxiety.

Panic attacks

Certain individuals get attacks of overwhelming panic, often for no obvious reason. Such attacks may occur as frequently as twice a week or, on the other hand, be very occasional. The attacks are characterised by a subjective feeling of terror related to a sensation of imminent death, together with pronounced tremulousness, profuse sweating and marked tachycardia. They usually occur in a public place and not unnaturally cause considerable alarm in those witnessing the attack. In most cases an ambulance is called and the patient rushed to hospital, but by the time he or she gets there the attack has abated considerably. If not, parenteral amylobarbitone (300 mg intramuscularly) or diazepam (10 mg intravenously) should calm the patient adequately.

When the attack has settled, long-term medication will often help in reducing the frequency of attacks; this should be as recommended for cases of moderate anxiety. In many of the patients, the attack begins with tachycardia; this frightens the patient into believing he is about to have a 'heart attack' which in turn exacerbates the tachycardia and leads in time to greater fearfulness. Beta-adrenergic blocking drugs may reduce the tendency to tachycardia and thus reduce the likelihood of a full-blown panic attack.

Situational anxiety and phobias

The term situational anxiety includes all the commonly recognised phobic symptoms. In addition, it includes those clinical states like psychogenic impotence and frigidity which are basically the result of anxiety confined to the sexual situation (see chapter 12).

Phobias often arise as the result of a learned experience. Unfortunately the lesson is learned too well and the patient becomes unable to accept the fact that he is unlikely to come to any further harm in the particular situation. There would appear to be three main categories of phobias: (1) specific phobias—a fear of spiders, a fear of heights (2) social phobias—a fear of meeting people or of eating in public (3) agoraphobia—a general fear of being away from the security of one's home.

In recent years it has come to be accepted that the most effective therapeutic approach to such conditions is behaviour therapy. This 'specific desensitisation' may take the form of gradually reintroducing the patient, at first in imagination, later, in reality, to his feared situation. Another technique 'implosion' or 'flooding' is to plunge the patient in at the deep end, as it were, by repeatedly confronting him with his most feared object or getting him to imagine himself in his most feared situation. Opinions remain divided on the most effective of the two methods but it appears that the implosive technique is better for agoraphobes, the great majority of whom fail to respond to specific desensitisation, while specific desensitisation works best in patients with specific phobias.

In both these treatments, psychotropic drugs are useful in producing the required reduction of central arousal for the relearning to take place. They can be prescribed as a long-term measure, for which a benzodiazepine is useful. In addition, the actual desensitisation or implosive procedure may be greatly facilitated by intravenous infusion of a rapidly metabolised barbiturate, methohexitone sodium (Brietal, Brevital) or a eugenol derivative, propanidid (Epontol) which is even more rapidly metabolised. These compounds are infused slowly intravenously during the course of a treatment session lasting up to thirty minutes. It is very important to avoid injecting too rapidly or the patient may be put to sleep. Furthermore it is absolutely necessary to have resuscitation apparatus at hand, together with a syringe charged with 1:1000 adrenaline before undertaking this treatment in case of an anaphylactoid reaction. Although both methohexitone and propanidid are equally effective, propanidid has the great practical advantage of causing less post-treatment drowsiness and a more rapid recovery. Even so, patients should be strongly discouraged from driving an automobile for several hours after a treatment session.

Apart from behaviour therapy, some recent studies have indicated that monoamine oxidase inhibitors, such as phenelzine (Nardil) 15 mg three times daily, may produce considerable improvement. While the rate of improvement with monoamine oxidase inhibition is quicker than with behaviour therapy, the tendency to relapse is much more marked with MAOI. As yet there have been few direct comparisons of MAOI with benzodiazepines in phobias; until such comparisons are undertaken, the exact place of MAOI in phobias must remain uncertain. Some authorities recommend gradually decreasing doses of benzodiazepines (beginning with intravenous diazepam in a 10 mg dose) together with gradual retraining; again whether or not this is better than MAOI treatment is undetermined.

Reports have recently appeared which indicate that the MARI drug, clomipramine (Anafranil) may markedly ameliorate phobic and obsessional symptoms.

Table 8   *Anxiolytic drugs*

Approved name	Proprietary name	Recommended dose (daily unless stated otherwise)	Remarks
benzodiazepines			
chlordiaze-poxide	Librium	10–100 mg	Effective anxiolytic compounds. Affect the limbic system before the cerebral cortex. Main advantage over barbiturates is in safety factor. Can produce dependence but less likely than barbiturates. Little to choose between individual members of this group
diazepam	Valium	4–80 mg	
oxazepam	Serenid-D Serax	20–90 mg	
medazepam	Nobrium	10–50 mg	
lorazepam	Ativan	3–10 mg	
clorazepate	Tranxene	15 mg	Administer once a day
barbiturates			
amylobarbitone sodium (UK) amobarbital (USA)	Sodium amytal	150–400 mg daily in divided doses or 1 hour before anxi-ety-provoking situation	Can lead to over-sedation. Over-dosage can be fatal; therefore use sparingly if any question of suicidal risk. Produces physical dependence, particularly in doses exceeding 1 g per day. Liver enzyme induction may occur
phenobarbitone (UK) phenobarbital (USA)	Luminal	150–400 mg	
propanediols			
meprobamate	Miltown Equanil	400–2400 mg	Rather weak anxiolytics. Developed from muscle-relaxants

Table 8—*Contd.*

tybamate	Benvil Solacen	500–1000 mg	More effective and with shorter half-life than meprobamate. Little if any advantage over benzodiazepines

diphenylmethanes

hydroxyzine	Atarax Vistaril	50–100 mg	Generally superseded by benzodiazepines
benactyzine	Suavitil		

neuroleptics

chlorpromazine	Largactil Thorazine	50–100 mg	Not as effective as barbiturates in anxiety
trifluoperazine	Stelazine	4–10 mg	Better than placebo. Not evaluated against benzodiazepines. Possibility of parkinsonian symptoms
haloperidol	Serenace	1–2 mg	No obvious advantage over benzodiazepines
oxypertine	Integrin	30–40 mg	As effective as benzodiazepines with possibly less psychomotor disturbance
pimozide	Orap	2–4 mg	Equal to benzodiazepines in efficacy. Administration required only once daily

Table 8—*Contd.*

Approved name	Proprietary name	Recommended dose (*daily unless stated otherwise*)	Remarks
monoamine reuptake inhibitor drugs			
doxepin	Sinequan	20–150 mg	Anxiolytic as well as anti-depressant. As effective as low-dose benzodiazepines but greater likelihood of autonomic effects
opipramol	Insidon Ensidon	100–150 mg	Tricyclic with piperazine side-chain. As effective as low-dose benzodiazepines
clomipramine	Anafranil	50–250 mg	Said to be of value in obsessional and phobic conditions
dibenzobicyclo-octadienes			
benzoctamine	Tacitin	20–100 mg	Equal in efficiency to benzodiazepines with similar sedative side-effects
miscellaneous			
fenfluramine	Ponderax	40–120 mg	Centrally sedating appetite suppressant of possible use in anxiety—particularly anxious obese patients
phenytoin (UK) diphenyl-hydantoin (USA)	Epanutin Dilantin	300 mg	Anticonvulsant shown to possess anxiolytic properties

Suggestions for further reading

General

LADER, M. H., 'Anxiety—new approaches' in *Topics in Therapeutics*, vol. 2, ed. P. Turner, Pitman, London, 1976.
LADER, M. H., *The Psychophysiology of Mental Illness*, Routledge & Kegan Paul, London, 1975.
LADER, M. H., BOND, A. J., and JAMES, D. C., 'Clinical comparison of anxiolytic drug therapy', *Psychological Medicine*, vol. 4, 1974, pp. 381–7.
LADER, M. H., and MARKS, I., *Clinical Anxiety*, Heinemann, London, 1971.
MARKS, I., *Fears and Phobias*, Heinemann, London, 1969.
TYRER, P., *The Role of Bodily Feelings in Anxiety*, Oxford University Press, London, 1976.

Benzodiazepines

BOND, A. J., JAMES, D. C., and LADER, M. H., 'Sedative effects on physiological and psychological measures in anxious patients', *Psychological Medicine*, vol. 4, 1974, pp. 374–80.
GARATTINI, S., MUSSINI, E., and RANDALL, L. O., *The Benzodiazepines*, Raven Press, New York, 1973.
GREENBLATT, D. J., and SHADER, R. I., *Benzodiazepines in Clinical Practice*, Raven Press, New York, 1974.
KESSON, C. M., GRAY, J. M. B., and LAWSON, D. H., 'Benzodiazepine drugs in general medical practice', *British Medical Journal*, vol. 1, 1976, pp. 680–2.
TYRER, P., 'The benzodiazepine bonanza', *Lancet*, vol. 2, 1974, p. 709.

Organic psychiatric syndromes

The term 'organic psychiatric syndromes' refers to those conditions in which there is a disturbance of psychological function due to a definite physical cause. That is not to say that other psychiatric conditions, such as schizophrenia or mania, are not primarily due to physical causes; they may well be. It is just that we have not yet determined with any confidence what they are (see chapters 6 and 7). In the case of the organic psychiatric syndromes, the disruption of cerebral function leading to the psychological disturbance may either be temporary (acute) or permanent (chronic).

Such phenomena as metabolic upsets, anoxia, hypoglycaemia, high fever and acute poisons frequently produce an impairment of cerebral function with an accompanying disturbance of consciousness. This gives rise to the clinical condition known as an 'acute confusional state'. Usually improvement of the underlying cause is followed promptly by amelioration of the mental state. In contrast, where the psychological impairment is due to permanent damage of the brain, as in *dementia* and the *dysmnesic syndrome* (see below), no significant spontaneous improvement can be expected.

Acute confusional state (delirium)

Whenever the level of consciousness is impaired, however slightly, there is an associated reduction in attention, with an increase in distractability. The more profound the reduction in consciousness the greater the psychological disturbance. This lessening of attention leads to a failure in grasping instructions and in registering new information. The patient thus becomes seemingly un-cooperative, even truculent. In addition there may be delusions of persecution, and these, together with the restlessness and irritability which commonly occur, can make nursing difficult. Inability to register new information leads to disorientation in time and space. Such disorientation together with clouding of consciousness are cardinal features of an acute confusional state.

Other symptoms include hallucinations, particularly visual hallucinations, dysphasia and perseveration, disconnected thinking; anxiety, sometimes amounting to frank terror, can also be present, particularly in delirium tremens (see below).

An acute confusional state can be caused by a wide variety of conditions; anything which interferes with brain function can bring it about. However, the clinical picture is largely the same whatever the pathogenesis; it is determined not so much by the primary cause as by: (i) the intensity and duration of the cerebral disturbance; (ii) the environmental stimuli present during the cerebral disturbance; (iii) the previous personality and experience of the patient.

Treatment must first be directed towards the underlying cause, and in many cases this will be sufficient to improve the psychological state. When rapid improvement of the basic disturbance is not possible, and the behaviour of the patient remains disturbed, then additional treatment specifically directed towards improving the mental state is usually indicated. In most cases cautious medication with chlorpromazine (Largactil, Thorazine) (see chapter 6) will suffice. As cerebral function is already impaired, and a lowered blood pressure accompanies many of the conditions producing an acute confusional state, it is essential to start treatment with a relatively small dose: 25–50 mg either orally or intramuscularly. If this does not produce the desired effect, and provided that there has been no worsening of the patient's clinical condition, the drug can be given subsequently in a larger dose: 50–100 mg. Occasionally it may be necessary to exceed 150 mg but this must be done with great care as most patients with an acute confusional state are already physically ill; adding what amounts to yet another toxic substance may well not improve matters overall.

In patients with liver failure the impaired detoxication of many anxiolytic sedatives and narcotics leads to an exaggeration and prolongation of their pharmacological effects; thus great caution must be exercised.

Delirium tremens

In contrast to other toxic confusional states, delirium tremens arises as a result of withdrawal of a drug (alcohol) rather than its administration. In order to reduce these withdrawal symptoms, which are very alarming and can even prove fatal, it is advisable to prescribe one of the benzodiazepine group of drugs, or chlormethiazole. Relatively large doses, given either orally or systemically are usually required for adequate sedation: chlordiazepoxide (Librium) 25–50 mg, diazepam (Valium) 20–40 mg or chlormethiazole (Heminevrin) 1·5–2 g are probably the drugs of choice (even larger doses than this may be needed in resistant cases). Some authorities still recommend intramuscular paraldehyde: 10–12 mg to start with, increasing up to 40 mg if necessary. In addition many patients are dehydrated and require rapid measures to correct their fluid balance. Finally, chronic alcoholism is often accompanied by a relative deficiency of thiamine and other B vitamins. Because of this, large doses of B vitamins are usually given systemically to patients with delirium tremens (see also chapter 10).

Dementia

Dementia, a condition characterised by a waning of intellectual powers, impairment of memory (particularly the retention of new information), emotional lability, a coarsening of the personality together with increasing disinterest in personal appearance and hygiene, comes about as a result of degeneration or destruction of the cerebral cortex. This may be caused by a variety of conditions, including hereditary degenerative diseases, the so-called pre–senile dementias (Huntington's chorea, Pick's disease, Alzheimer's disease, Creutzfeld–Jacob's disease), trauma, toxic substances (lead and mercury), metabolic disturbance (prolonged hypoglycaemia, myxoedema), pernicious anaemia, infections (particularly syphilis), and neoplasms. However, more common than any of the above are cerebral arteriosclerosis and 'senile' degeneration, both occurring much more frequently in the elderly. Recent surveys have revealed that of those aged sixty-five or over about 5 per cent are suffering from frank dementia and another 5 per cent are suffering from a milder form. The great majority in both categories are living in the community, institutional care being provided for relatively few. Approximately half of these individuals are suffering from cerebral degeneration secondary to arteriosclerosis; the other half have senile dementia. Before considering any drug treatment (see below) close attention should always be paid to providing adequate social and personal support.

Arteriosclerotic dementia

Dementia due to cerebral arteriosclerosis tends to run a fluctuating course. In addition, there are usually focal neurological signs together with a raised blood pressure. Post-mortem studies reveal widespread areas of cerebral softening. The greater the degree of intellectual impairment present the greater the total area of cerebral softening found. Unfortunately, treatment of established arteriosclerosis is largely unavailing; certainly by the time dementia has occurred no measures designed to alter such factors as the general blood pressure level are likely to do much good. However, some claims have been made for cyclandelate (Cyclospasmol), isoxsuprine (Duvadilan) and dihydroergotoxine (Hydergine) which appear to increase cerebral blood flow; improvement in intellectual capacity and memory has been reported after a few months continuous treatment with cyclandelate 400 mg four times daily. Unfortunately, there appeared to be no correlation between the degree of improvement in cerebral circulation observed with radio-circulograms and the level of improvement in psychometric test scores. Furthermore, the ward nursing staff failed to note any greater improvement in the patients given cyclandelate as compared to those given placebo. A more recently introduced compound naftidrofuryl (Praxiline) has proved superior to placebo in controlled trials. However, until more comprehensive studies have been completed, the place of these drugs in the treatment of arteriosclerotic dementia must remain uncertain, and their routine use in the elderly showing mental impairment has not yet been justified. Treatment of associated disturbed behaviour is as for senile dementia (see below).

Senile dementia

In many respects senile dementia can be seen as a gross exaggeration of the normal ageing process, although whether the two differ qualitatively as well as quantitatively is an open question. From the pathological point of view, they would appear to differ only in degree, rather than kind. Normal ageing is associated with the appearance of so-called senile plaques (argentophil plaques) in the cerebral cortex. In senile dementia there are many more such plaques, and the greater the number of plaques the more severe the dementia. In contrast to arteriosclerotic dementia, the course is continuous and there are few, if any, focal neurological signs. There may be a family history of senile dementia, and it is this genetic predisposition which leads some authorities to consider that senile dementia is distinct from normal ageing. It has been suggested that the histological changes noted in senile dementia are so similar to those found in Alzheimer's disease that the two conditions should be treated as one, with senile dementia being considered as Alzehimer's disease coming on in later life. Neurochemically there would also appear to be a similarity; within the cerebral cortex, hippocampus and the amygdala the levels of choline acetyltransferase and acetylcholinesterase have been found to be reduced. These enzymes are involved in the metabolism of the neurotransmitter acetylcholine and it might be that the pathogenesis of this condition is related to a failure in the cholinergic system in the brain.

Neurophysiologically there is often a slowing in the frequency and in the amount of the alpha rhythm in the EEG. There is also a slowing of conduction time in peripheral nerves, as well as a significant increase in latency in the EEG-recorded somatosensory evoked response. These findings suggest that the basic disturbance in senile dementia may be a generalised slowing of conduction within the nervous system.

There is no known treatment which effectively reverses or even halts the underlying pathological process. Controlled trials of a wide variety of substances including folic acid, androgenic hormones and procaine hydrochloride (substance 'H') have shown them all to be quite ineffective. Many patients, particularly in the later stages of the disease, exhibit disturbed behaviour both during the day and in the night. The most suitable drug for daytime control is thioridazine (Melleril) in a dose of 25–100 mg given up to three times daily. While extrapyramidal symptoms are less likely with this drug than with other phenothiazine compounds, there is a risk of retrolental fibroplasia and of retinitis if a daily dosage of 600 mg is continued for more than a few months. A suitable alternative drug is haloperidol 0·5–6 mg daily, but here the risk of extrapyramidal reactions is greater; should these occur an antiparkinsonian agent may be required in addition (see chapter 6).

For night sedation chloral hydrate given as syrup or as dichloralphenazone (Welldorm) 650–1300 mg is suitable (see chapter 11).

Barbiturates should be avoided. Other possible alternatives include nitrazepam (Mogadon) 5–10 mg and chlormethiazole (Heminevrin) 0·5–1.0 g in tablet form; in many cases the syrup form may prove more acceptable; up to 20 ml may be required.

Dysmnesic syndrome (Korsakoff's psychosis)

Although profound memory disturbance occurs in acute confusional states and in dementia, it is but a part, albeit an important part, of a much wider disturbance of psychological function. The term 'dysmnesic syndrome' refers to those cases in which there is a considerable impairment in the cerebral mechanism underlying the process of remembering without any clouding of consciousness (as in acute confusional state) and without any general deterioration in intellect (as in dementia). Most commonly the dysmnesic syndrome follows Wernicke's encephalopathy, itself a consequence of chronic alcoholism. When this happens the condition is synonymous with Korsakoff's psychosis; there are, however, other possible causes including encephalitis, trauma, tumours of the third ventricle and carbon monoxide poisoning.

In the dysmnesic syndrome the major defect is in the retention of new information. Patients can recognise new information perfectly well, and are able to repeat it for a period of a few minutes afterwards. Yet, within a relatively short time they have no recollection of it whatsoever. The consolidation of new information into the memory store is completely blocked. Although the biochemical and physiological basis for memory is as yet ill-understood, there is greater knowledge regarding the anatomy. Bilateral lesions limited either to the mammillary bodies (as in Korsakoff's psychosis) or to the hippocampus are sufficient to produce the full clinical picture of the dysmnesic syndrome.

The inability to retain new information results in patients becoming disoriented in time and space so that they may not remember such things as the day of the month or where they are. Many patients realise their deficiencies in this regard and when pressed will invent answers to fill the gaps (confabulation). Such confabulation is, however, not an essential component of the syndrome. It has been suggested that long-term memory storage is associated with subtle alterations of chemical substances within the brain. As ribose nucleic acid (RNA) was thought to be involved, attempts have been made to provide extra RNA to patients with the dysmnesic syndrome in the hope of improving their capacity to remember. Thus far the results of such attempts have been equivocal, and any improvement noted did not appear to be permanent. While administration of thiamine is unlikely to affect any marked change in memory it should be given a trial either parentrally or orally, particularly in the early stages (see chapter 10).

Huntington's chorea

This is an hereditary condition, transmitted by an autosomal dominant gene with each child of an affected patient standing a 50:50 chance of developing the disease. As it does not normally come before the third or fourth decade, there is a considerable risk that a genetically predisposed individual will have fathered or borne children before knowing they were going to get it themselves. Typically choreiform movements precede the onset of a progressive dementia.

Histologically, there is marked atrophy of the caudate nucleus and putamen. Recent neurochemical studies have indicated that the neurotransmitter gamma-aminobutyric acid (GABA) and its biosynthetic enzyme, glutamic acid decarboxylase, are significantly reduced in the globus pallidus, the substantia nigra, the caudate nucleus and the putamen. The finding that GABA receptors are intact would imply that treatment with GABA-mimetic drugs might prove useful in modifying the choreiform movements, although they would not be likely to influence the course of the progressive dementia. Unfortunately, treatment with sodium valproate (Epilim), a compound found to elevate brain GABA in animals by inhibiting glutamate transaminases, has thus far proved disappointing. The loss of the inhibiting action by GABA on dopaminergic (DA) neurones (see chapter 2) may result in an increased DA effect. In keeping with this, phenothiazine compounds, which block DA receptors, currently afford the best available treatment. Thioridazine (Melleril) 50–150 mg or tetrabenazine (Nitoman) 25 mg two or three times daily are probably the most generally useful drugs in the management of Huntington's chorea.

Suggestions for further reading

BERGMAN, K., 'The epidemiology of senile dementia', in *Contemporary Psychiatry*, ed. T. Silverstone and B. Barraclough, *British Journal of Psychiatry* Special Publication, no. 9, 1975.

BIRD, E. D., and IVERSEN, L. L., 'Neurochemical findings in Huntington's chorea', in *Essays in Neurochemistry and Neuropharmacology*, vol. 1, ed. M. B. H. Youdim, W. Lovenberg, D. F. Sharman and J. R. Lagnado, John Wiley, Chichester, 1977.

CORSELLIS, J. A. N., 'The pathology of dementia', in *Contemporary Psychiatry*, ed. T. Silverstone and B. Barraclough, *British Journal of Psychiatry* Special Publication, no. 9, 1975.

CRAMOND, W. A., 'Organic Psychosis', *British Medical Journal*, vol. 4, 1968, pp. 497–500.

DAVIES, P., and MALONEY, A. J. F., 'Selective loss of central cholinergic neurones in Alzheimer's disease', *Lancet*, vol. 2, 1976, p. 1403.

DRUG AND THERAPEUTICS BULLETIN, 'Drugs for dementia', vol. 13, 1975, pp. 85–7.

LEVY, R., 'The neurophysiology of dementia', in *Contemporary Psychiatry*, ed. T. Silverstone and B. Barraclough, *British Journal of Psychiatry* Special Publication no. 9, 1975.

LISHMAN, W. A., 'Amnesic syndromes and their neuropathology', in *Recent Developments in Psychogeriatrics*, ed. D. W. K. Kay and A. Walk, *British Journal of Psychiatry* Special Publication no. 6, 1971.

MCLELLAN, D. L., CHALMERS, R. J., and JOHNSON, R. H., 'A double-blind trial of tetrabenazine, thiopropazate and placebo in patients with chorea', *Lancet*, vol. 1, 1974, pp. 104–7.

IO   Personality disorders, alcoholism and drug dependence

The personality of an individual refers to that special combination of psychological traits which make him the particular person he is. It can be considered in much the same way as his physical constitution, which again is a unique amalgam of anatomical and physiological features.

While we can accurately measure such anatomical features (e.g. height), we are far less able to quantify the various personality traits. We are even uncertain about the number of traits involved. Nevertheless, personality theorists generally agree that the following are among the more important characteristics: neuroticism (anxiety-prone); obsessionality (meticulous); tendency to hysterical behaviour (self-centred, histrionic); psychopathy (antisocial); extraversion/introversion; reliability; independence.

All of us exhibit these traits to some degree; where we differ from one another is in the quantity, rather than the quality, by which they are expressed.

Personality traits can best be considered as continuous rather than discrete variables. For instance we are all somewhat prone to be anxious (i.e. neurotic); but, while some people are made anxious by the least disturbance in the environment, others hardly turn a hair, even in what to many would be a most alarming situation. The majority feel anxious in what would be generally accepted as anxiety-provoking circumstances such as examinations, job interviews and public performances. It is only when anxiety becomes extreme, or occurs under minimal stress, that treatment is indicated (see chapter 8).

Similarly, social conformity varies from one person to another: at one extreme is the self-sacrificing, saint-like person, at the other is the selfish, inconsiderate bully. It is this latter group to which the term *psychopath* or sociopath generally refers. Psychopathy is but one of the so-called personality disorders (character disorders). Others include: (1) the hysterical personality (self-centred, histrionic and unreliable); (2) the dependent personality (unable to function independently, weak, easily led); (3) the obsessional personality (extremely meticulous and conscientious); (4) the explosive personality (unpredictable, given to violent outbursts); (5) the paranoid personality (suspicious, always ready to take offence); (6) the schizoid (introvert) personality (introspective, shy, sometimes aloof and emotionally cold); (7) the anxiety-prone (neurotic) personality (worries about everything). It is only when the abnormality of personality causes actual suffering to the individual concerned, or to society in general, that the term 'disorder' is justified.

Unfortunately, treatment has relatively little to offer in terms of 'cure'. Indeed, the very concept of cure is misconceived in this group of patients; we might just as well speak of 'curing' someone with an IQ of 70. All we can do is to help the patient get along with the psychological constitution (personality and intelligence) he has. Certainly by the time adulthood is reached, there is little, if any, hope of significantly influencing personality; we cannot turn the chronic worrier into a devil-may-care sort of fellow, nor can we easily transfer the callous psychopath into a model citizen. We may, however, through a psychotherapeutic approach, allow the patient to appreciate how his (or her) personality tends to produce or exacerbate certain situations, and how he or she affects other people. In addition, newer behavioural techniques offer great promise in this direction.

As far as drug-treatment is concerned, the possibilities are limited. We may afford symptomatic relief to the anxiety-prone individual, and to some degree to the chronic hypochondriacs, with anxiolytic-sedative drugs of the benzodiazepine type (see chapter 8). Other personality disorders are less amenable to drug treatment. Although claims have been made that pericyazine or propericiazine (Neulactil), a phenothiazine derivative, effectively reduces violent antisocial behaviour in those of a psychopathic personality, the claims are largely unsubstantiated by controlled experiments, and should, therefore, be accepted with caution.

Severe obsessional symptoms may be helped by administration of a monoamine reuptake inhibiting drug (MARI) (see chapter 7). A member of this group of drugs, clomipramine (Anafranil), has been specifically tested for its ability to alleviate obsessional disorder. Administration may be intravenous (up to 250 mg clomipramine in normal saline or 5 per cent dextrose infused over a period of one to two hours), or oral, 75 to 450 mg daily in divided doses. Although initial results appear encouraging, enthusiasm must be tempered until results from more double-blind studies are reported.

Finally, certain patterns of abnormal behaviour, including sexual deviation, alcoholism and drug dependence, are reflections of an underlying personality disorder. The place of drug treatment in the management of sexual deviation is discussed in chapter 12, while alcoholism and drug dependence are considered in the following sections of this chapter.

Alcoholism

An alcoholic may be defined as an individual who causes problems for himself, or creates difficulties for others, by reason of excessive drinking. Although the detailed pattern of alcohol consumption may vary from patient to patient, no resolution of these problems and difficulties is likely to take place without a drastic overall reduction of alcohol intake. Alcoholism is extremely prevalent in most Western societies; in the UK the estimated total number approaches half a million. The situation in the USA is even worse; there, according to some authorities, about five million can be described as alcoholics, at an annual cost to the community of over a billion dollars.

The exact place of drug treatment in this condition has not yet been clearly established. It would appear to be of considerable benefit in the withdrawal phase, of probable benefit in some patients as a deterrent to further drinking, and of possible benefit in reducing the desire for alcohol in abstinent ex-alcoholics.

Withdrawal symptoms

When someone who has been regularly consuming large quantities of alcohol suddenly stops drinking altogether, he may well experience withdrawal symptoms, which are a consequence of physical dependence on the drug. These can vary from mild nausea, tremulousness, headaches and general malaise to frank delirium tremens.

When mild, these symptoms usually require little more than a period of rest, together with one of the benzodiazepine drugs, either chlordiazepoxide (Librium) 10–25 mg or diazepam (Valium) 5–10 mg three times daily; an equally effective alternative is chlormethiazole (Heminevrin) 1–1·5 g two or three times daily.

In contrast, the serious condition of frank delirium tremens calls for much more vigorous treatment. Clinical management includes the recognition and treatment of any concurrent medical condition, and the maintenance of an adequate fluid balance. In some cases emergency measures to counter profound hypothermia or severe hypotension may be necessary; in any case a regular watch must be maintained on temperature, pulse and blood pressure.

Treatment of the delirium itself is with large intramuscular doses of chlordiazepoxide, up to 50 mg on the first day, followed by an oral dose of up to 25 mg four times daily. Diazepam is equally effective. Paraldehyde can be given, up to 10 mg every four hours on the first day, and every six hours on the second day, followed by 20 mg at night on subsequent days. A third suitable alternative is chlormethiazole, given in an initial dose of up to 2 g.

As many patients who have reached this stage in their condition have long-standing nutritional deficiencies, it is not unreasonable to administer large doses of high-potency vitamins systemically, although it should be appreciated that there is no evidence to suggest that vitamins are in any way a specific remedy for delirium tremens.

Deterrence from further drinking

Quite by chance, two doctors who had been taking disulfiram (Antabuse) in the course of an investigation into its possible use as an antihelminthic, experienced a series of extremely unpleasant physical reactions after attending a cocktail party. They were quick to conclude that the drug they had been taken had inter-fered with their metabolism of alcohol thus producing a toxic reaction; disulfiram by itself had produced no such ill-effects. As a result of this observation, disulfiram was given to selected alco-holics, who although they wished to stop drinking lacked the necessary resolve to persevere. They knew that if they drank after taking disulfiram they would experience marked ill-effects, due to the presence of acetaldehyde in their circulation. The serum acetaldehyde level rises because disulfiram competes with the acetaldehyde formed from the metabolism of alcohol for the enzyme acetaldehyde dehydrogenase. The competitive inhibition of this enzyme causes the blood level of acetaldehyde to rise, producing a syndrome characterised by widespread vasodilatation, (causing a violent throbbing sensation), vomiting, chest pain and dyspnoea. In addition there is a pronounced fall in blood pressure, leading to vertigo, blurred vision, and eventual collapse. The rationale behind such treatment is the hope that, in order to avoid the acetaldehyde syndrome, an alcoholic will desist from drinking once he has taken his daily disulfiram. As long as he continues to take it the potential effect will remain; however, if the patient stops taking his daily disulfiram, within a week all its effects will have worn off, and he will feel no symptoms of the acetaldehyde syndrome no matter how much he may drink. Unfortunately, this approach helps only that relatively small proportion of alcoholics whose resolve is sufficient to ensure regular administration of their disulfiram, but who without their deterrent might weaken during the course of the day. Some intrepid patients even 'drink through' their acetaldehyde reaction, potentially a highly dangerous procedure. Because of this possibility patients must be very carefully selected before being placed on a disulfiram treatment programme.

It is no longer considered necessary to submit the patient to a preliminary test with disulfiram, or citrated calcium carbonate (see below), plus alcohol; such a procedure carries considerable risk. After an initial loading dose, a maintenance dose of disulfiram of one tablet containing 0·2 g daily is sufficient for most patients.

Although disulfiram by itself was originally thought to be without ill-effect, experience has revealed that depression, malaise, bad-breath (due to a garlic-like flavour), impotence, gastrointestinal symptoms, and occasionally peripheral neuropathy may be produced by the drug, particularly at a dose level higher than 0·5 g per day. Because of these effects many patients are reluctant to persist in taking disulfiram for a sufficient length of time, and consequently relapse. There is also evidence that it may influence the anticoagulant activity of warfarin and interfere with prothrombin control.

As an alternative, a citrated calcium carbimide (Abstem, Temposil) which produces similar effects in combination with alcohol has the advantage of being much more rapidly metabolised and thus less likely to produce unwanted side-effects. The required dose is 50–100 mg per day.

The reduction of craving

Claims have been made that metronidazole (Flagyl) significantly reduces the craving for alcohol experienced by many alcoholics. While the earlier enthusiastic reports were not substantiated by relatively short-term controlled trials, the results from a recent twelve-month study indicated that patients taking metronidazole regularly in a dose of 600 mg daily did better than patients on placebo; 31 per cent or more in the active drug group were classified as 'improved' after twelve months compared to 3·5 per cent of those in the placebo group. It is thought that the drug acts by reducing anxiety, and by altering the taste of alcohol. The use of such an approach is somewhat limited, for patients who conscientiously persist in taking medication for such a relatively long period are hardly typical of alcoholic patients as a whole.

Therefore, while long-term drug therapy of either the deterrent type or the metronidazole type may help some alcoholics, the great majority require repeated or continuous psychological and social support; the part which drugs can play in the long-term management of this condition is at present very limited.

Finally, it should not be forgotten that some individuals are what might be considered symptomatic drinkers; that is, they drink excessively only when they become depressed as part of an affective disorder or develop symptoms of acute anxiety. In every case of alcoholism an attempt should be made to recognise any such precipitating factors; if present they should be treated promptly. Alleviation of any underlying depression (see chapter 7) or anxiety state (see chapter 8) will often reduce the patient's need to consume the alcohol which he had previously required for relief of his psychological distress.

Treatment of neurological complications

1 Wernicke's syndrome of ataxia, diplopia and confusion requires urgent treatment with replacement thiamine. Parenteral administration of 50 mg thiamine daily is recommended until the clinical state has improved sufficiently, when oral administration can be substituted.

2 The dysmnesic syndrome (Korsakoff's psychosis), (see chapter 9), which may occur in long-standing alcoholism, is less responsive to thiamine replacement, but its onset may be prevented by early

and adequate thiamine replacement whenever there is evidence of diplopia or of cerebellar signs.

3   Alcoholic polyneuropathy should be treated with a combination of thiamine, pantothenic acid, nicotinic acid and pyridoxine, as deficiencies of all these substances are thought to play a part in the pathogenesis of the neuropathy. Treatment should continue for several months as resolution of symptoms can be slow.

Drug dependence

Psychological and, in many instances, physiological dependence on drugs is an ever-increasing problem in our society, particularly among the young. Drug dependence is by no means limited to 'hard' drugs like heroin and cocaine, or to illegal drugs like cannabis. Numerically there is a much larger problem of dependence on commonly prescribed preparations containing stimulants of the amphetamine type, or anxiolytic sedatives such as barbiturates.

Drug dependence has been defined by the World Health Organisation as:

A state, psychic and sometimes also physical, resulting from the interaction between a living organism and a drug characterised by behavioural and other responses that always include a compulsion to take the drug on a continuous or periodic basis in order to experience its psychic effects and sometimes to avoid the discomfort of its absence. Tolerance may or may not be present. A person may be dependent on more than one drug.

Some further WHO definitions of the terms used are as follows:

Tolerance: 'the phenomenon of dose increase to maintain the drug effect'.
Physical dependence: 'an adaptive state that manifests itself by intense physical disturbances when the administration of the drug is suspended or when its action is affected by the administration of a specific antagonist'.
Psychic dependence: 'the intense craving and compulsive perpetuation of abuse to repeat the desired effect of a psychotropic drug'.

Drugs likely to lead to dependence all have in common the property of producing a rapid heightening of mood, or reduction of tension, followed by a feeling of 'let-down', which in turn can only be relieved by taking more of the drug.

Clinical features of dependence vary with the drug in question, and can best be considered individually in relation to the groups of compounds causing dependence, namely: (1) drugs of the morphine type (2) drugs of the barbiturate type (3) drugs of the amphetamine type (4) drugs of the cocaine type (5) drugs of the cannabis type (6) hallucinogenic drugs.

While the pattern of dependence may vary with the drug, the personality of the individual who becomes dependent tends to be similar. The most frequent type of personality observed in a patient presenting with drug dependence can broadly be described as 'inadequate'; he is often someone who cannot cope with the normal frustrations of life without some form of psychological prop. Such a person usually requires immediate gratification, finding any delay intolerable, with a consequent tendency to impulsive and ill-considered behaviour. There are, of course, many people with similar characteristics who are not drug-dependent, but the addict has found or selected a particular way, namely the use of centrally acting drugs, of coping with his emotional problems and gratifying his psychological needs. It should be noted that not all addicts show this characteristic personality structure, and social and environmental factors play a large part in determining the occurrence and the pattern of drug abuse and drug dependence.

1 *Dependence on drugs of the morphine type* As was mentioned in the Introduction, the use and abuse of opiates dates from pre-history, but it was not considered a social problem until the eighteenth century. At that time the East India Company exploited the addictive properties of opium commercially, and this in turn led to the opium wars in the next century. Following the introduction of injectable morphine into military medicine during the American Civil War, a number of soldiers became dependent, a condition referred to at the time as the 'soldier's disease'. Heroin, originally produced as a non-addictive alternative to morphine, proved itself an even greater menace and most opiate addicts in Western society now take heroin, usually intravenously.

During the period up to the 1950s heroin dependence in the UK was largely confined to therapeutic addicts, i.e. patients who had originally been prescribed heroin or morphine for some medical condition. The remainder were doctors or nurses who had ready access to the drug.

More recently the pattern of heroin dependence has changed, with far more young 'non-therapeutic' addicts being introduced to drug taking by their friends. The total number of heroin addicts in the UK is approximately 2,000 (just over twenty-five per million); in the USA the prevalence is over ten times as great with an estimated 56,000 heroin addicts (290 per million). In neither country is the problem quite so alarming as it is in Iran, where there are thought to be 50,000 opium addicts (6,550 per million) or Hong Kong with its 11,000 addicts (2,900 per million). Not only is the pattern and degree of addiction different in the two countries but the laws of each also show marked differences. Although heroin prescription in the UK is limited to authorised doctors working in drug-dependency clinics, addicts are allowed, and even encouraged to be treated on an out-patient basis obtaining strictly regulated supplies of heroin from their local pharmacist—in the USA it is illegal to prescribe heroin to addicts outside certain specified in-patient facilities under any circumstances, or for any individual to possess heroin. American addicts consequently resort to crime in order to obtain enough money to buy their supplies illegally and drug dependence has become inextricably bound up with criminality in the USA.

An addict's first experience of heroin is often during a weekend jaunt with friends, one of whom is already dependent and who encourages the other to inject himself. The first few injections may be subcutaneous but these soon give way to intravenous injections ('mainlining') which gives a more immediate sensation ('buzz'). At first, heroin injections will be limited to occasional weekend use, but self-injection soon becomes more frequent until, within a matter of months, the addict is no longer injecting heroin for positive pleasure; he is desperately trying to avoid the unpleasant effects accompanying withdrawal. These include shivering with pilo-erection (hence the term 'cold-turkey'), watering of the eyes and running nose, abdominal cramp followed by vomiting and diarrhoea. Individuals vary considerably in the intensity with which such symptoms are experienced.

Perhaps the most disturbing aspect of heroin dependence is the high mortality of young, previously healthy, adults and adolescents. The mortality rate is twenty times that of non-addicts, and is due largely to secondary infection accompanying intravenous injections without sterile precautions, rather than to the direct action of the drug itself, although in some cases death follows an accidental overdose.

Treatment is aimed at withdrawal and abstinence, either gradually on an out-patient basis, or rapidly in an in-patient unit. Recent experience at the special drug-dependency clinics in the UK indicates that the former approach is likely to be more successful in the long term, particularly if accompanied by an accepting, supportive attitude on the part of all concerned.

2   *Dependence on drugs of the barbiturate type*   This is probably the most widespread, but least-recognised form of drug dependence, apart from alcoholism. Some 80,000 people are overtly dependent on barbiturates in the UK (this is equivalent to over 0·2 per cent of the adult population) and ten times that number take a regular small amount of barbiturates; some six million prescriptions for barbiturates are issued each year.

Although reports of barbiturate dependence appeared in the 1920s the seriousness of the situation was not realised until relatively recently.

The great majority of cases were prescribed barbiturates as hypnotics either as part of hospital routine when they happened to be in-patients, or by their general practitioners. Cerebral activity is affected by even brief exposure to hypnotics. Cessation of the drug leads to a rebound disturbance of sleep with increased restlessness and dreaming, and the patient, trying to overcome these symptoms, reverts to the sleeping tablet he has been trying to do without.

Unlike other drugs of dependence, many more women than men are dependent on oral barbiturates. Intravenous use, which has recently become more prevalent, is largely confined to young people who include barbiturates in their pattern of polydrug abuse. Increasing doses are required to offset tolerance and the characteristic picture of ataxia, nystagmus, dysarthria and drowsiness should alert one to the likelihood of barbiturate intoxication in a previously normal woman.

Serious withdrawal symptoms may occur after stopping barbiturates, particularly if the daily intake has been in excess of 1 g per day. These may include an episode of frank delirium punctuated by epileptic convulsions.

As with other drug dependency problems, withdrawal and subsequent abstinence are the therapeutic goals. In view of the serious nature of the withdrawal symptoms it is best carried out in hospital where gradual reduction of barbiturate intake can be attempted.

Doctors have a particular responsibility in preventing dependence on barbiturates; and in general they should no longer be prescribed for either anxiety or insomia.

3 *Dependence on drugs of the amphetamine type* Soon after the introduction of amphetamine in the early 1930s its stimulant and euphoriant properties became widely recognised, and amphetamine abuse created clinical and social problems within a very short time. By the 1950s the contents of amphetamine inhalers were being extracted on a large scale and ingested by young people in the UK, Scandinavia, the USA, and Japan. When the availability of such inhalers was restricted, interest turned to amphetamine in tablet form, either alone or in combination with barbiturates (Drinamyl, 'Purple Hearts'). In recent years the use of injectable methylamphetamine (methedrine, 'speed') has become widespread. However, since its distribution in the UK was restricted to hospitals, there has been a gratifying reduction in its abuse.

Two quite distinct groups of people become dependent on amphetamine. First there are the otherwise relatively stable, often middle-aged women for whom amphetamine is prescribed to help them lose weight (see chapter 13); they seek repeated small doses of amphetamine to avoid the lethargy they experience when they are without the drug. The second group are much more emotionally unstable young adults or adolescents who take ever-increasing amounts to attain a state of euphoria and to ward off fatigue. As the effects wear off they experience a profound depression which can only be satisfactorily relieved by further amphetamine. Abuse in this group may lead to restlessness and irritability, resulting in unreasoning aggression towards others. On examination the pupils are dilated and there is a rapid pounding pulse. If amphetamine is taken over a long period a marked weight loss occurs.

Amphetamine psychosis can follow a number of large doses (50 to 100 mg) taken over a relatively short time. In this condition the patient is tormented by vivid auditory hallucinations and paranoid delusions. In some ways amphetamine psychosis resembles an acute schizophrenic episode but unlike schizophrenia the symptoms promptly wane when the drug is withheld.

As no physical dependence to amphetamine occurs, treatment is by simple withdrawal, although the possibility of a serious post-drug depressive state must be guarded against. Adequate social rehabilitation and psychological support will usually be required.

In the view of most medical authorities, amphetamines have little place in clinical practice, apart from narcolepsy and the hyperkinetic syndrome in children (see chapter 15).

4 *Dependence on drugs of the cocaine type* Cocainism, still a problem in South America, is becoming less prevalent in the developed countries where its use is largely confined to heroin addicts who take it to offset the sedative effects of heroin. Although heroin dependence remains as serious as ever most addicts, in the UK at least, no longer find it so necessary to add cocaine, and many drug-dependency centres are not prepared to prescribe it.

Cocaine, like amphetamine, is a central-nervous stimulant producing no physical dependence. When taken in large doses it leads to a state of over-activity and excitement, which may be accompanied by a most uncomfortable sensation in the skin reminiscent of insects crawling all over one's body (formication).

5 *Dependence on drugs of the cannabis type* Probably no drug in recent times has been surrounded by more controversy and contention than cannabis, the mixture of substances obtained from the unfertilised flower heads of Indian hemp. There are at least four pharmacologically active substances in the resin: (i) tetrahydrocannabinol (THC) which depresses acetylcholine release within the intestine (ii) a second closely related substance (iii) a fat-soluble central-nervous depressant (iv) a water-soluble atropine-like substance.

It is difficult to know exactly what the psychopharmacological effects of cannabis are, as the subjective experiences vary so much with the social conditions under which it is taken. Regular users report a hazy glow of contentment, accompanied by a sharpening of perception and heightened sense of appreciation, particularly of jazz music; in contrast, naive users often find that the effects, if any, are somewhat unpleasant. It produces little in the way of physiological effects apart from a rise in heart rate and a reddening of the conjunctiva. On psychological testing, cannabis was found to impair psychomotor performance in naive smokers but not in regular users.

High dosage can result in frank delirium and associated paranoid delusions followed by subsequent amnesia for the whole episode.

6 *Dependence on hallucinogenic drugs*   We have already noted how preparations, like mescaline, with hallucinogenic properties can become incorporated into religious rites (see chapter 1). More recently, particularly since the development of remarkably potent synthetic hallucinogens like lysergic acid diethylamide (LSD), the ingestion of hallucinogens has spread to other societies, partly in the belief that they may be therapeutic, and partly in the hope that the perceptual experiences produced will widen artistic horizons.

The amounts of LSD required to produce psychological effects are minuscule, as little as one millionth of a gram per kilogram body weight being sufficient, and of this, only one per cent actually crosses the blood brain barrier.

LSD produces autonomic, sensory and emotional effects, in that sequence, over the course of some twelve to twenty-four hours. The autonomic effects include gastrointestinal activity leading to vomiting and diarrhoea, pupil dilation, pilo-erection and tremor. Following these there is a dramatic alteration of visual perception which allows the subject to perceive the world in a quite extraordinarily novel way. It is this distortion of perception which has so attracted to LSD certain intellectuals and artists who hoped to find a new stimulus to creativity through the drug. At the same time, or shortly afterwards, there is an awareness of a change in the quality of experience, which has been described in such terms as 'ecstatic', 'mystical', 'transcendental', but, as with many other drugs, these effects depend to a considerable degree on the social situation in which LSD is taken and the expectations of those taking it. Unfortunate sequelae to LSD can occcur, particularly when the sensation of power and invulnerability displaces all caution. Under such conditions subjects may jump off buildings in the conviction that they cannot possibly come to harm. The LSD experience ('trip') may also give way to depression and consequent suicide.

The illicit use of LSD is confined to a few and the prevalence of regular users in the UK is probably less than one per 100,000. It is unlikely to have a useful place in psychiatric treatment.

Treatment of dependence on opiate drugs

While drug treatment plays a relatively minor part in the overall management of this condition (in the UK at least), it is of considerable use when dealing with withdrawal symptoms. Furthermore the substitution of oral methadone for intravenous diamorphine (heroin) has been widely advocated as the best way of coping with the situation, although the considerable disadvantages of substituting one narcotic for another are becoming more generally recognised. A third area in which drug treatment may be of some limited use is in the maintenance of abstinence, although continued social and psychological support is likely to be of more lasting value.

The management of withdrawal

In the recently established treatment centres in Great Britain drug withdrawal is a gradual process usually undertaken under outpatient conditions. Under these circumstances there is no appearance of the classical withdrawal symptoms: lacrimation, rhinorrhoea, yawning, pilo-erection and perspiration; proceeding to extreme restlessness, violent cramp-like pains, retching and vomiting, accompanied by tachycardia and raised blood pressure. However, when the drug is stopped abruptly, then the clinical picture of withdrawal, as just described, is not only extremely distressing, but it may prove harmful also, and requires urgent treatment. Pharmacologically, the withdrawal symptoms can be terminated by administration of the drug to which the patient is addicted, but in most situations this is unlikely to be desirable, even if possible. A compound which has a similar pharmacological spectrum to heroin, such as methadone (Physeptone), can be given orally at a starting dose of 20–30 mg. This is often given with diazepam 10–20 mg. Over the next few days the dose of methadone can be reduced by 20 per cent per day, with only minimal symptoms of withdrawal.

Psychological factors play a large part in the manifestation of the withdrawal syndrome and a supportive reassuring approach can often itself greatly reduce the severity of the symptoms experienced.

An alternative regime employs a combination of diphenoxylate and atropine (Lomotil) together with chlormethiazole (Heminevrin). The diphenoxylate, which is a congener of pethidine, reduces the physical symptoms while the chlormethiazole relieves any anxiety the addict may feel regarding withdrawal. Dosage is as follows: diphenoxylate 2·5 to 5·0 mg (1–2 tablets of Lomotil) and chlormethiazole 1·0 to 2·0 g (2–4 tablets of Heminevrin) four hourly throughout the working day plus nitrazepam (Mogadon) 10 mg at night if required.

Should a heroin addict appear in a doctor's surgery (office) or hospital casualty department (receiving room) showing clear physical withdrawal symptoms, he should be given methadone up to 20 mg orally and be watched while he takes it. Arrangements can then be made for him to attend an appropriate treatment centre within the next twenty-four hours.

A situation in which withdrawal symptoms may present a serious threat to life is in babies born to opiate-dependent mothers. The first signs may appear before delivery as foetal distress. Should this occur it is imperative to ensure that the mother receives sufficient opiate to counter the withdrawal symptoms in the foetus. After delivery the infant suffering from withdrawal symptoms usually presents with irritability and tremulousness, which may be accompanied by vomiting and diarrhoea, as well as yawning, sneezing, respiratory distress, excess mucous secretion and even convulsions. Prompt treatment with chlorpromazine, 1 mg/kg body weight every four hours, is essential. This dose may be reduced over the course of the next few days.

Drug substitution

As it remains a crime to prescribe heroin in many countries, including the USA, medical authorities have turned to methadone as a drug which they can prescribe, and which the addict can obtain, without committing a felony. Whereas in Great Britain licensed doctors in specified treatment centres are able to prescribe heroin (albeit with stringent safeguards), American doctors cannot do this. Therefore, in the USA the addict is faced with the choice of getting heroin illegally (which demands an enormous, unceasing financial outlay often supported by criminal activities) or methadone legally. Unfortunately, substitution of one narcotic for another hardly affects the underlying problem; it merely reduces the need for the addict to indulge in criminal acts in order to pay for the drugs he needs.

Methadone substitution as practised in the USA consists of administering a daily oral dose of methadone. The addict is frequently required to attend the clinic daily to obtain this medication, which lasts him throughout the twenty-four-hour period, until he is due for his next dose. Recent studies have indicated that while withdrawal effects may be expected forty-eight hours after a methadone-free period, the effects of a new derivative, l-α-acetylmethadone last longer, and administering acetylmethadone three times a week should prove as effective as methadone daily.

Another situation where regular methadone administration is useful occurs when an addict, maintained on intravenous heroin during the day, finds that as the effect of his evening dose does not last throughout the night he gets restless in the early hours. Here a methadone mixture, up to 20 mg at night, with its greater duration of action, will usually afford a good night's sleep.

Narcotic antagonists

Substitution of an allyl group for the N-methyl group in morphine and morphine-like substances often leads to antagonism of the parent group of compounds. For instance nalorphine hydro-bromide (Lethidrone) and nalorphine hydrochloride (Nalline) which are n-allyl morphine salts and naloxone (Narcan) which is n-allyl-diamorphine are potent morphine and heroin antagonists. When nalorphine, 1–3 mg is administered subcutaneously to someone who has recently taken a substantial dose of a narcotic drug, acute withdrawal symptoms will be experienced within fifteen minutes; these reach a peak within an hour, and persist for at least two hours. It has been suggested that the narcotic antagonists act by competing for receptor sites within the body. Cyclazocine has a similar mode of action.

These substances have been used in the supportive treatment of abstinent ex-addicts in much the same way as disulfiram is used in alcoholism. The abstinent ex-addict is advised to take daily cyclazocine 4–6 mg daily; he then knows that if he subsequently takes heroin or methadone he will experience withdrawal symptoms. Unfortunately, as with disulfiram in alcoholism, only a minority of the patients, who are insufficiently motivated to maintain abstinence without any drug, are sufficiently conscientious in their self-medication to persist for long enough. Naloxone, 0·4 mg intravenously, is often valuable in the management of overdosage of narcotic analgesics (see chapter 16).

Suggestions for further reading

Alcoholism

CALDWELL, J., and SEVER, P., 'The biochemical pharmacology of abused drugs II. Alcohol and barbiturates', *Clinical Pharmacology and Therapeutics*, vol. 16, 1974, pp. 737–49.

DRUG AND THERAPEUTICS BULLETIN, 'Treatment for neurological complications of alcoholism', vol. 11, 1973, pp. 85–7.

DRUG AND THERAPEUTICS BULLETIN, 'The management of alcoholism', vol. 12, 1974, pp. 77–9.

EDWARDS, G., 'The meaning and treatment of alcohol dependence', in *Contemporary Psychiatry*, ed. T. Silverstone and B. Barraclough, *British Journal of Psychiatry* Special Publication, no. 9, 1975.

GLATT, M., *The Alcoholic and the Help he Needs*, 2nd edn, Priory Press, London, 1972.

Drug dependence

BEWLEY, T. H., 'An introduction to drug dependence', in *Contemporary Psychiatry*, ed. T. Silverstone and B. Barraclough, *British Journal of Psychiatry* Special Publication, no. 9, 1975.

CALDWELL, J., and SEVER, P. S., 'The biochemical pharmacology of abused drugs, III. Cannabis, opiates and synthetic narcotics', *Clinical Pharmacology and Therapeutics*, vol. 16, 1974, pp. 989–1013.

CANADIAN GOVERNMENT COMMISSION OF INQUIRY: Interim Report, *The Non-Medical Use of Drugs*, Penguin, Harmondsworth, 1971.

CONNELL, P. H., *Amphetamine Psychosis*, Chapman, London, 1958.

GHODSE, A. H., 'Drug dependent individuals dealt with by London casualty departments', *British Journal of Psychiatry*, vol. 131, 1977, pp. 273–80.

OSWALD, I., 'Dependence upon hypnotic and sedative drugs', in *Contemporary Psychiatry*, ed. T. Silverstone and B. Barraclough, *British Journal of Psychiatry* Special Publication, no. 9, 1975.

PATON, W. D. M., 'Cannabis and its problem', *Proceedings of the Royal Society of Medicine*, vol. 66, 1973, pp. 718–21.

WORLD HEALTH ORGANISATION, Report of the Expert Committee on Addiction-producing Drugs, *World Health Organisation Technical Reports Series*, no. 273, 1964.

Sleep disturbance 11

Nature of sleep

Although sleep is an activity which occupies about one third of our life, its nature is still poorly understood. The notion that sleep is a state analogous to suspended animation, a state of cellular inactivity, was exploded when electroencephalographic records taken during sleep showed persistent electrical activity, but of a different character to that seen in the waking state. Furthermore, experiments in which subjects have been woken at frequent intervals have suggested that some sort of mental activity can go on all through the night, but that it is almost entirely, if not completely, forgotten on waking.

The timing of sleep in the rhythm of the day's activity is learnt rather than inborn. The sleep of newborn babies tends to be regulated more by their feeding schedule than by the clock. After this early period of life, however, sleep, in common with other factors such as body temperature and diuretic activity, is governed by a twenty-four-hour rhythm. This in turn probably depends on the effects of alteration of light and darkness on hypothalamic centres which then influence hormonal activities in other parts of the body through the pituitary gland. Fast air travel across the world has emphasised the importance of our learnt diurnal sleep rhythm. Many travellers find that it takes them several days to adjust their sleeping habits when they make journeys across the Atlantic or further afield.

Even if some mental activity continues during sleep, there is no doubt that a sleeping person is in a state of inertia, being unresponsive to outside events, and that a large part of the mental activity which occurs is forgotten on waking. Electroneurophysiological studies in animals have shown that the reticular formation in the brain stem is intimately concerned with the state of consciousness and responsiveness. When the reticular formation is destroyed, leaving intact the main sensory pathways to the cerebral cortex, animals are in a perpetual sleep, confirmed by the EEG, even though sensory impulses from the periphery still reach the cortex. When, on the other hand, sensory tracts to the cortex are divided above their afferent branches to the reticular formation, the animals sleep at intervals, but may be awakened by a stimulus such as noise. They waken spontaneously and are fully active between their sleep periods. If *consciousness* implies an awareness of a recognised stimulus and the ability to respond to it, then this is not possible without a cerebral cortex, and these latter animals cannot be said to be conscious. *Wakefulness*, however, is not the same as consciousness and is possible without a cerebral cortex. It is primarily dependent on the functional integrity of the reticular system.

Electrical activity of the brain in normal sleep may be divided into two phases. The first is characterised by large-amplitude, low-frequency waves at one to three cycles per second in which sleep is profound ('slow wave sleep', 'orthodox sleep'). Brief bursts of faster activity at about twelve cycles per second are generally mixed in with these slow waves and are known as 'sleep spindles'.

The second phase, which occurs at intervals between periods of orthodox sleep, consists of low-amplitude, high-frequency, 'sawtooth' waves, accompanied by rapid conjugate movements of the eyes ('activated sleep', 'dream sleep', 'paradoxical sleep', 'rapid eye movement—REM sleep'). Respiration, heart rate and blood pressure are irregular and the penis may be erect during this phase. If subjects are wakened while their EEG record shows evidence of REM sleep activity, they usually report that they were dreaming vividly. This phase occupies in all about a quarter of the total night's sleep, recurring about five times during the night. When wakened during orthodox sleep they are more likely to report 'thinking' without emphasis on imagery, action or emotion.

Electroneurophysiologists have further divided orthodox sleep into four stages. Stage 1 is the lightest phase in which subjects are most easily wakened. As sleep deepens, the EEG waves become slower and larger, reaching a maximum in Stage-4 sleep which appears the most intense and from which it is most difficult to rouse the subject. Stages 3 and 4 occur mainly in the early part of the night, and are most apparent in subjects who have been deprived of sleep. It has been suggested that orthodox sleep is associated particularly with general tissue restoration, as athletes tend to have more Stage-3 and 4 sleep on nights after strenuous physical exercise. Furthermore, secretion of human growth hormone is increased in Stage-3 and 4 sleep, no output occurring in the absence of these stages. This hormone promotes protein synthesis, and peaks of mitotic activity in skin, bone, marrow, liver and the reticulo-endothelical system occur at this time. REM sleep, on the other hand, has been related to synthetic and restorative functions in the brain, because of the increase in cerebral blood flow which accompanies it, and because of its association with the neonatal period when brain growth is rapid; it appears proportionately less in mental defect and in senility, when synthetic processes in the brain are impaired.

Hypnotism

Despite widespread misconceptions to the contrary, a subject in a so-called hypnotic trance is not asleep. Many studies have shown that the pulse and respiration rate, blood pressure, cerebral blood flow and skeletal muscle reflexes are all characteristic of the waking rather than sleeping state. These observations are confirmed by the EEG which shows a waking record.

Effects of drugs on sleep

A large number of drugs influence sleep. Central-stimulant compounds, such as caffeine, theobromine, amphetamine and its derivatives, produce varying degrees of insomnia with a reduction in total duration of night sleep, while central-depressant compounds such as barbiturate drugs induce sleep and prolong its duration. The effects of centrally acting drugs on the electrophysiological phases of sleep are more complex, however. Both central stimulant and depressant compounds reduce the proportion of time spent in REM sleep. Therapeutic doses of pentobarbitone, amphetamine, phenmetrazine, methylphenidate, tranylcypromine and diethylpropion all reduce the proportion of the time spent in REM sleep to between 14 and 18 per cent of total sleeping time. Alcohol, too, depresses REM sleep in normal subjects. Combinations of a barbiturate with amphetamine, for example in the proprietary preparation 'Drinamyl', produce an even more marked reduction in REM sleep than either constituent alone. When these centrally acting drugs are withdrawn after chronic administration there is a rebound period during which there is an increased proportion of the night spent in REM sleep, particularly at the beginning of the night. Oswald has suggested that suppression of REM sleep and the rapid appearance, upon withdrawal, of REM sleep rebound are characteristic of drugs which lead to dependence and abuse. He has also suggested that the slow return of brain function to normal as measured by the EEG sleep pattern, which may take up to five or six weeks after withdrawal of a hypnotic drug, indicates that protein synthesis is required for the reformation of neuronal 'machinery' altered by the drug during the period of adminstration.

The role of neurotransmitter substances in producing various stages of sleep is still uncertain and the evidence conflicting. Non-specific reduction of brain 5HT and noradrenaline levels in animals by reserpine reduces both orthodox and REM sleep. Parachlorophenylalanine, a selective inhibitor of 5HT synthesis, markedly decreases REM sleep in man, while orthodox sleep remains either unchanged or is slightly increased. This is in contrast to its effects in other mammals in which orthodox sleep is decreased. Monoamine oxidase inhibitors, such as tranylcypromine, which increase tissue concentrations of 5HT and noradrenaline, lead to a progressive reduction in REM sleep and increase in orthodox sleep, both in man and experimental animals. Intracerebral or intraventricular injections of 5HT or 5HTP in animals similarly lead to an increase in the time spent in orthodox sleep at the expense of REM sleep. Although these studies appear to implicate 5HT in the regulation of sleep, other investigations have suggested that REM sleep can be initiated or sustained by cholinergic drugs, and can be blocked or reduced by anticholinergic drugs, and stimulated by noradrenaline or its precursor dopa. Gamma-aminobutyric acid and certain short-chain fatty acids also induce sleep when injected parenterally under suitable conditions.

Further experiments in man in which l-amphetamine was found to be equipotent to d-amphetamine in suppressing REM sleep suggest that noradrenaline (NA) as well as 5-HT might be involved in REM sleep. This suggestion arises on the basis that l-amphetamine and d-amphetamine are equipotent in suppressing neuronal reuptake of NA, whereas d-amphetamine is 3–4 times as potent as l-amphetamine in suppressing dopamine (DA) reuptake. On the other hand, as d-amphetamine has a greater effect than l-amphetamine on total sleep time and on wakefulness generally, it is likely that DA is concerned with that aspect of sleep.

Prolonged hypnotic effects and hangover

An ideal hypnotic drug should not only induce sleep rapidly and predictably and maintain sleep for a reasonable length of time without influencing the ratio of orthodox to REM sleep, but it should also be free from prolonged central effects. In most comparative studies of hypnotic drugs, the incidence of persistent 'hangover' effects has been assessed retrospectively and without objective tests to confirm their duration. In recent years, however, investigations have been carried out into the duration of central depression produced. Quinalbarbitone 200 mg given at bedtime was found to impair performance in a battery of psychological tests up to fifteen hours later. In other studies, nitrazepam 5 and 10 mg, and amylobarbitone sodium 100 and 200 mg were studied thirteen hours after administration to subjects who abstained from central stimulants such as caffeine. Although the subjects considered themselves alert, behavioural and psychomotor tests showed significant impairment. Further investigations showed that hypnotic doses of nitrazepam or a barbiturate impaired performance twelve hours after administration, even if subjects were allowed their usual intake of coffee or tea. These results are not surprising when it is considered that the half-lives of barbiturate hypnotic drugs and nitrazepam are between ten and twenty hours in most subjects. Flurazepam, however, has a shorter half-life and as such should be less prone to cause residual effects. This was found to be true of the 15 mg dose when given to patients for whom the drug was being prescribed for insomnia, but not true for normal volunteer subjects, nor for a 30 mg dose in either patients or volunteers. It is obviously important when hypnotic drugs are prescribed to warn patients of the probability of diminished efficiency on the following day, particularly in relation to driving and other skills. EEG changes due to hypnotic drugs persist very much longer than impairment of psychomotor function.

Withdrawal of hypnotic drugs

Few responsible people would dissent from the view that dependence on hypnotic drugs is undesirable and that the present increase in such dependence should be reversed. Where possible, patients dependent on these drugs should be weaned off them, but it appears that this process should be carried out gradually rather than abruptly. The sudden withdrawal of hypnotic drugs produces a 'rebound' increase in REM sleep and recent investigations have suggested that some organic disease states, such as angina and myocardial ischaemia, gastric hyper-acidity and peptic ulceration, may be exacerbated during periods of increased paradoxical sleep. Caution should be exercised, therefore, in withdrawal of hypnotic drugs in patients with coronary artery disease or a history of peptic ulceration. Furthermore, abrupt withdrawal of barbiturates and occasionally of the benzodiazepines, can lead to convulsions.

Treatment of insomnia

Difficulty in sleeping is an extremely common complaint, as witnessed by the vast numbers of various sorts of sleeping tablets prescribed. It is estimated that some 600 million tablets or capsules are taken annually in the UK while the consumption in the USA is ten times as great. Of increasing importance is the frequency with which overdosage from sedative drugs occurs. With these factors in mind it should hardly be necessary to emphasise how important it is to avoid over-enthusiastic medication for what is, after all, a condition which itself carries no risk.

Before deciding on a course of treatment it is necessary to determine the causes of the sleep disturbance. Basically these are of four types:

(i) Secondary to some other condition producing discomfort, adequate treatment of which is the obvious first approach.
(ii) Environmental change in working patterns, or rapid shift from one time-zone to another as occurs in long-distance air travel. Shift workers who have to adjust to sleeping during the day one week, only to revert back to nocturnal sleeping the following week, may find it difficult to go to sleep for a night or two after changing shifts. Here, cautious and limited use of a hypnotic preparation is not unreasaonable. A similar approach can be used for those travellers who may take a little while to adjust their diurnal rhythm to their new surroundings.

Another common environmental cause is having to sleep in strange surroundings, particularly in hospital, where an unfamiliar bed, the general unease felt by most when in hospital, and the noise made by other patients, all combine to prevent a good night's sleep. This is of course well recognised by medical and nursing staff. Some may consider that it is rather too well recognised in that it has become almost standard practice to prescribe night-time sedation for all patients before it is known whether or not they require it. Such practice is potentially harmful as many former patients become chronically dependent on sleeping tablets as a direct result of having first been given them while in hospital.

(iii) Certain illnesses are characterised by sleep disturbance which is an integral part of the condition. The most common such condition seen in psychiatric practice is depressive illness (endogenous depression), where early morning wakening is frequent. Patients describe how, although they can go to sleep without too much trouble, they waken in the early hours of the morning and are unable to go to sleep again. Their depression is often particularly severe at this time and the risk of suicide consequently high. It has been suggested that this change in the sleeping pattern may be related to the changes in ACTH secretion which occur in depressive illness with the morning peak coming some two to three hours earlier than normal.

Although hypnotic drugs may help to relieve the early morning wakening, treatment of the underlying depressive illness will obviously be the first step in management (see chapter 7).

(iv) By far the most common cause of sleeping difficulty is worry or emotional strain: mothers worried about their children, husbands concerned over their job, adolescents crossed in love. All can lie awake, tossing and turning, brooding over their problems.

Eventually they nearly always get off to sleep, but do not feel refreshed when they waken to face their problems again. In many such cases frank discussion of their fears and worries may itself relieve the tension sufficiently to render any pharmacological intervention unnecessary.

Before any prescription for sedative drugs is given to a patient, he should be warned against the possible synergistic effects of alcohol, and should be cautioned against drinking shortly before, or after, taking his night sedation.

Finally, doctors should be sparing in the quantity of tablets or capsules prescribed at one time, thus minimising the risk of overdosage; similarly, they should be cautious in the frequency with which they prescribe hypnotic drugs to any one patient, thus minimising the risk of dependence. It has been shown that counselling patients about the possibilities of dependence when initially prescribing a hypnotic, and closely monitoring repeat prescriptions, can markedly reduce the likelihood of patients becoming dependent on these compounds.

Choice of therapy

Although there is a bewildering array of hypnotic drugs, in practice the most widely used fall into three main categories: benzodiazepines, barbiturates and chloral hydrate derivatives.

1 *Benzodiazepines* As has been stated previously (chapter 8) all the marketed benzodiazepine compounds are potential hypnotics if given in sufficient dosage. Two benzodiazepines, flurazepam (Dalmane) and nitrazepam (Mogadon), have been specifically marketed as hypnotics. Nitrazepam would appear to have no obvious advantage over diazepam, and if insomnia presents a problem in a patient for whom diazepam is indicated during the day there is no reason to use another benzodiazepine at night, instead a final dose of diazepam can be taken before retiring. However, when insomnia is the sole symptom, and treatment with a hypnotic appears indicated, then the drug of choice is flurazepam in a starting dose of 15 mg one hour before retiring. A number of controlled trials have attested to its efficacy, and its shorter half-life makes it preferable to nitrazepam.

2 *Barbiturates* Barbiturates have generally fallen into disfavour as hypnotics because of their tendency to produce liver enzyme induction (see chapter 3) and even more because of the much greater danger associated with over-dosage as compared to benzodiazepines. Furthermore they are very likely to cause confusion in the elderly.

Among the barbiturates there is very little to choose from among those listed in Table 9. They all have more or less the same duration of action and all require to be taken in approximately the same dosage. In most cases 100 mg taken one hour before retiring will be sufficient, although in some patients, particularly where anxiety is intense, 200 mg may be required. There is no advantage to be gained from a mixture of barbiturates, or from a mixture of other drugs with a barbiturate. Where reliable trials have been conducted into the efficacy of such mixtures, it has invariably been found that it is the barbiturate content which counts.

3 *Chloral hydrate* This is a relatively weak hypnotic which, when absorbed, is metabolised to trichlorethanol. Its main disadvantage is its unpleasant taste and it also has an unfortunate tendency to produce gastric irritation. It should therefore be taken well-diluted with milk or olive oil. The preparation, dichloralphenazone (Welldorm), which is in tablet form, may be a more acceptable way of administering the same compound, being particularly useful in the elderly.

Continuous sedation

Some psychiatrists find that continuous sedation, or 'sleep treatment', may be of value in severe, prolonged anxiety states although, the efficacy of this approach has never been rigorously tested. The aim is to keep the patient asleep for the greater part of the day over a period of several days. Large doses of barbiturates (200–300 mg three or four times a day) are required, and skilled nursing care is needed to prevent respiratory complications or pressure sores. Physical dependence on barbiturates can occur if the treatment goes on long enough and withdrawal fits can provide an added complication.

Narcolepsy

In this condition, the pathogenesis of which remains obscure, patients are frequently overtaken by irresistible attacks of sleep from which they can be readily wakened. Attacks, which may occur several times in one day, are characteristically brought on in susceptible individuals by emotional arousal. Narcolepsy is probably the only condition in adults for which administration of amphetamine is justified. It can be given either as the racemic mixture amphetamine sulphate (Benzedrine) or as the dextrorotatory-isomer, dexamphetamine sulphate (Dexedrine), both in a dosage of 5–10 mg three or four times a day. Methylphenidate (Ritalin) 10–20 mg two to four times daily is an effective alternative. Milder degrees of narcolepsy may respond to caffeine, either given as tablets (100–300 mg), or taken in coffee.

Table 9 *Hypnotics*

Approved name	Proprietary name	Recommended dose	Remarks
benzodiazepines			
nitrazepam	Mogadon	5–10 mg	Effective and relatively safe although likely to produce hangover effects
flurazepam	Dalmane	15–30 mg	
barbiturates			
amylobarbitone sodium (UK) amobarbital (USA)	Sodium Amytal	100–200 mg	Well tried, effective hypnotics. Can produce confusion in the elderly and drug dependence in the susceptible. Over-dosages frequently fatal. Not too much to choose between them. All relatively cheap
butobarbitone (UK) butobarbital (USA)	Soneryl	100–200 mg	
heptabarbitone (UK) heptabarbital (USA)	Medomin	200 mg	
pentobarbitone (UK) pentobarbital (USA)	Nembutal	50–100 mg	
quinalbarbitone (UK) secobarbital (USA)	Seconal	50–100 mg	
quinalbarbitone and amylobarbitone	Tuinal	100–200 mg	No advantage over its constituents prescribed singly
carbromal (and pento- barbitone 100 mg)	Carbrital	250 mg	Efficacy almost entirely attributable to barbiturate content
chloral hydrate derivatives			
chloral hydrate trichlorethyl phosphate	Somnos Triclofos	1–2 g well-diluted	Safe, particularly useful in the elderly. Unpleasant taste with tendency to produce gastric irritation

Table 9—*Contd.*

Approved name	Proprietary name	Recommended dose	Remarks
dichloral-phenazone	Welldorm	650–1300 mg	Relatively weak hypnotic, useful in elderly
others			
ethchlorvynol	Arvynol Serenesil Placidyl	250–500 mg	Equally effective as barbiturates and glutethamide. Seems safe and relatively cheap
ethinamate	Valmid	500 mg	Short-acting. Useful for initiating sleep. Little hangover effects
glutethimide	Doriden	250–500 mg	Although classified as non-barbiturate efficacy and side-effects similar. May be excreted more rapidly with less prolonged effects
meprobamate	Equanil, Miltown	400–800 mg	Good in the elderly
methaqualone (and diphen-hydramine 25 mg)	Quaalude Mandrax	150–300 mg 250 mg	Moderately effective Rapid onset of action. Considerable tendency to produce dependence. Over-dosage difficult to treat
methyprylone	Noludar Noctan Dimerin	200–300 mg	Actions and toxic effects similar to chloral hydrate

Suggestions for further reading

Sleep and its disorders

FENTON, G. W., 'Clinical disorders of sleep', *British Journal of Hospital Medicine*, vol. 14, 1975, pp. 120–45.

HAURI, P., 'Sleep in depression', *Psychiatric Annals*, vol. 4, 1974, pp. 45–62.

LANCET, Editorial, 'Sleep', *Lancet*, vol. 1, 1975, p. 963.
OSWALD, I., 'Sleep difficulties'. *British Medical Journal*, vol. 1, 1975, pp. 557–8.
OSWALD, I., 'The function of sleep', *Postgraduate Medical Journal*, vol. 52, 1976, pp. 15–18.
PARKES, J. D., 'The sleepy patient', *Lancet*, vol. 2, 1977, pp. 990–3.
RATNA, L., 'The psychophysiological aspects of dreaming', *British Journal of Hospital Medicine*, vol. 9, 1973, pp. 203–10.

Neurochemistry of sleep

FENTON, G. W., 'The neurophysiological aspects of sleep', *Postgraduate Medical Journal*, vol. 52, 1976, pp. 5–9.
HARTMAN, E., and CRAVENS, J., 'Sleep: effects of d- and l-amphetamine in man and rat', *Psychopharmacology*, vol. 50, 1976, pp. 171–5.
JOUVET, M., 'Neurophysiological and biochemical mechanisms of sleep', in *Sleep*, ed. A. Kales, Lippincott, Philadelphia, 1969.

Hypnotic drugs

BARRACLOUGH, B. M., 'Are there safer hypnotics than barbiturates?', *Lancet*, vol. 2, 1974, pp. 57–8.
CLIFT, A. D., 'Factors leading to dependence on hypnotic drugs', *British Medical Journal*, vol. 3, 1972, pp. 614–17.
GREENBLATT, D. J., SHADER, R. I., and KOCH-WESER, J., 'Flurazepam hydrochloride', *Clinical Pharmacology and Therapeutics*, vol. 17, 1975, pp. 1–14.
JOHNS, M. W., 'Sleep and hypnotic drugs', *Drugs*, vol. 9, 1975, pp. 448–78.
KALES, A., BIXLER, E. O., SCHARF, M., and KALES, J. D.. 'Sleep laboratory studies of flurazepam: a model for evaluating hypnotic drugs', *Clinical Pharmacology and Therapeutics*, vol. 19, 1976, pp. 576–83.
MALPAS, A., LEGG, N. J., and SCOTT, D. F., 'Effects of hypnotics on anxious patients', *British Journal of Psychiatry*, vol. 124, 1974, pp. 482–4.

Residual effects of hypnotic drugs

BOND, A. J., and LADER, M. H., 'Residual effects of hypnotics', *Psychopharmacologia*, vol. 25, 1972, pp. 117–32.
MALPAS, A., ROWAN, A. J., JOYCE, C. R. B., and SCOTT, D. F., 'Persistent behavioural and electroencephalographic changes after single doses of nitrazepam and amylobarbitone sodium', *British Medical Journal*, vol. 2, 1970, pp. 762–4.
SALKIND, M. R., and SILVERSTONE, T., 'A clinical and psychometric evaluation of flurazepam', *British Journal of Clinical Pharmacology*, vol. 2, 1975, pp. 223–6.

Sexual problems

Physiology of sexual behaviour

The study of human sexual function can best be considered under two headings: drive and performance.

Sexual drive

The drive towards sexual activity has both strength and direction, and is largely under the control of the central nervous system. While the strength of sexual drive can be markedly influenced by physiological and pharmacological factors, the direction it takes in man is almost entirely determined by psychological and social influences.

In contrast, the direction of sexual behaviour of lower mammals is markedly influenced by pituitary function. For instance, in the guinea pig an injection of testosterone into the developing foetus will lead to a male type of behaviour pattern in later life, whatever the gonadal sex. In rats similar effects can be obtained with testosterone injection up to fifteen days post-natally. On the other hand oestrogens have no such effects. It is therefore considered that it is the absence of androgens in the females of lower mammalian species, rather than the presence of oestrogens, which directs psychological development into characteristic female behavioural patterns. In humans, however, social factors play a much more dominant part in determining gender role. For instance, female infants born with a hyperactive adrenal gland, and a consequently high androgen level (the adrenogenital syndrome), may be confused with a male at birth, particularly because the over-developed clitoris may be mistaken for a penis. If adequate steroid therapy is instituted to reduce pituitary ACTH secretion, the adrenal androgen levels fall and normal feminisation takes place, although there may be a persistent tomboyish tendency. There seems to be little indecisiveness in subsequent gender identification and no tendency towards homosexuality in spite of the high pre-natal androgen levels, which in lower animals would have had a lasting effect. Similarly, males with pronounced hypospadias, leading to a mis-classification of gender, can develop either in the male or the female role, after plastic repair. The important thing is for the parents to be consistent in their attitude.

At puberty, development of secondary sex characteristics is dependent on gonadal activity which in turn is influenced by the pituitary. Castrated males (eunuchs) fail to develop sexually and have limited sexual interest. Replacement therapy with androgens leads to normal sexualisation and an increase in the strength of sexual drive. Stopping such medication results in a diminished ejaculatory volume, fewer erections and less sexual desire. In con-trast the sexuality of females with hypogonadism is little impaired and not at all influenced by oestrogen replacement, although certain women with reduced libido may be helped by androgens (see below). Thus in both sexes it is the androgens which influence the strength of the sexual drive, but not the direction this drive will take.

Primate females undergo a regular monthly cyclic change in their output of oestrogens and progesterone, corresponding with the menstrual cycle. These fluctuations in hormone levels may in some cases be accompanied by changes in sexual responsiveness. Certainly in rhesus monkeys the sexual activity reaches its maxi-mum at mid-cycle when ovulation occurs. This has obvious bio-logical advantages: with the gradual fall followed by a short-lived rise in oestrogen, and the steady rise followed by a sharp pre-menstrual drop in progesterone concentration which takes place in the second, or luteal, phase of the menstrual cycle, sexual activity falls. This not only directly affects the female's responsiveness, but also impairs the attractiveness of the female for the male monkey, as measured by the number of mounting attempts. Similarly, the administration of oral contraceptive preparations containing 1 mg ethynodiol diacetate and 0·05 mg mestranol to female monkeys leads to a gradual reduction in the number of ejaculations by the male. These findings suggest that at least two mechanisms underlie sexual responsiveness in monkeys. First, there is an oestrogen-dependent vaginal change which stimulates the male, probably through his sense of smell. Second, there is an oestrogen action on the central nervous system of the female, which increases her responsiveness. This view has been substantiated by ingenious conditioning experiments where it was found that oophorectomised females were not a reward for male monkeys until they had been given oestrogens.

Many human females also notice a similar waxing and waning of sexual desire during the menstrual cycle, although here the picture is more complex. For instance, oophorectomy appears to have but little effect in human sexual activity in contrast to monkeys. Nevertheless, hypophysectomy does lead to a profound fall in the level of sexual desire and satisfaction, probably due to the secondary reduction in the level of adrenal androgens. Thus, in humans, sexual behaviour takes place in response to both internal (physiological) and external (psychological and social) factors, the actual behaviour pattern being largely determined by genetic predisposition and previous experience.

It is believed that hormones may influence the activity of neuro-transmitter amines. For example testosterone has been found to reduce the turnover of 5-hydroxytryptamine (5HT), and it may be that reduction of 5HT activity is the basis of the positive effect of androgens on sexual drive. In keeping with this view is the finding, albeit in lower animals, that reduction of brain 5HT caused by parachlorophenylalanine (PCPA) will strikingly increase the sexual behaviour of rats and of rabbits. It may be that dopamine (DA) is also involved in the regulation of sexuality in a way reciprocal to 5HT; DA precursors such as levodopa, and DA agonists such as apomorphine, can induce sexual behaviour in rats. These presumed DA effects are in turn abolished by DA receptor blocking drugs such as haloperidol, although this only applies to the initiation of sexual activity; once it has started DA-receptor blockade has little effect.

In women relative hypothalamic-pituitary DA insufficiency, as manifest by hyperprolactinaemia, which is often accompanied by reduced sexual drive, may be reversed by the DA agonist bromocriptine.

Human sexual performance

Until Masters's and Johnson's recent comprehensive observations of human sexual performance under laboratory conditions, knowledge of the detailed physiological changes which take place during sexual intercourse was poorly understood. According to Masters and Johnson, the human sexual response in both sexes occurs in four more or less distinct phases: the excitement phase, the plateau phase, orgasm and, finally, resolution.

These will now be discussed for each sex separately.

Sexual performance of the male

1 *Excitement phase*   This phase is characterised by penile erection. The penis consists of three cylindrical bodies of erectile tissue, which receive their blood supply from the internal pudendal arteries. When these arteries and their arterioles dilate, under the control of parasympathetic splanchnic nerves, blood fills trabeculated cavernous spaces within the erectile tissue and erection occurs. On contraction of the arterioles, under the control of the sympathetic nerves accompanying the arteries, the penis becomes flaccid.

Excess sympathetic activity, as occurs in anxiety states, will prevent penile erection and thereby hinder satisfactory sexual intercourse. Similarly malfunction or malformation of the parasympathetic nerve supply may also be a rare cause of failure of erection. Once a man has failed to obtain or maintain a satisfactory erection, the next time he attempts intercourse he is likely to be worried that he will fail. The very fact of his worrying tends to further increase sympathetic activity and prevent satisfactory penile erection. A vicious circle develops leading to the clinical condition of impotence.

2 *Plateau phase*   After the erection of the penis there is an increase in tumescence.

3 *Orgasm phase*   Just before orgasm a slight mucoid emission occurs which can contain motile spermatozoa. This may be a result of secretion from Cowper's glands. Almost immediately the vasa efferentia, the epididymis, the vasa deferentia, the seminal vesicles and the prostate all contract and together with the perineal muscles propel the seminal fluid rapidly through the penile urethra to the external meatus.

4 *Resolution phase*   This refers to the period following orgasm before the individual is ready to commence intercourse again. The duration of this period can vary considerably.

Sexual performance of the female

1 *Excitement phase* The first physiological manifestation of sexual arousal in women is the moistening of the vaginal walls from a transudation of fluid from the plexus of veins surrounding the vagina. It is not a true secretion, as there are no glandular elements within the vaginal wall.

Shortly afterwards there is vasocongestion of the breasts and nipple erection, engorgement of the labia majora and labia minora, and some distention of the clitoris.

2 *Plateau phase* This phase is marked by a localised vasocongestion of the outer third of the vagina which later contracts strongly during orgasm.

3 *Orgasm phase* Masters and Johnson describe this phase as 'a brief episode of physical relief from the myotonic and vasocongestive increment developed in response to sexual stimuli'.

4 *Resolution phase* This tends to be of much shorter duration than in the male.

In both males and females the cycle of sexual response described is possibly developed from 'a drive of biologic-behavioural origin deeply integrated into the condition of human existence'. There is, however, marked variation in the intensity and duration of the sexual response, which is to a large degree affected by social and psychological influences. Sexual fears in the female tend to be concerned either with the attainment of satisfactory orgasm or the sexual drive in general, whereas in the male sexual fears have related almost entirely to the attainment and maintenance of a penile erection. Not surprisingly perhaps, pharmacological remedies have long been sought for these problems.

Drugs affecting sexual behaviour

Sexual desire and performance may, as we have seen, be affected by psychological factors like anxiety, by the level of circulating androgens, by the activities of the autonomic nervous system and by local stimulation of the genital tract. Drugs influencing these functions may thus have an effect on sexual behaviour.

Although from time immemorial men have sought love philtres

to arouse the passion of women and to increase their own sexual powers, it is only in recent times that attempts have been deliberately made to reduce sexual drive. Furthermore, certain centrally acting drugs used in psychiatry have the disturbing property of adversely affecting sexual performance. Also with the advent of oral contraceptives many women have noted a profound effect of these compounds on their sexuality. Each of these topics will be considered in turn.

Drugs to increase sexual drive and performance (aphrodisiacs)

Centrally acting psychotropic drugs

1 *Anxiolytic sedatives* Anxiolytic sedatives and alcohol, by reducing subjective anxiety, may lower the level of sympathetic discharge sufficiently to allow penile erection to occur in cases of impotence. The dosage is critical, however, for too high a blood level may itself inhibit the parasympathetic mechanism controlling the blood supply to the penile erectile tissue. Shakespeare's summary of this pharmacological action of alcohol can hardly be bettered:

Lechery, sir, it provokes, and unprovokes: it provokes the
desire, but takes away the performance: therefore much
drink may be said to be an equivocator with lechery: it makes
him and it mars him; it sets him on, and it takes him off; it
persuades him and disheartens him; makes him stand to, and
not to stand to; in conclusion, equivocates him in a sleep, and,
giving him the lie, leaves him.   (*Macbeth*, Act II, Scene 3)

Frigidity in women is often due to an irrational anxiety about sexual intercourse. Allaying such anxiety with anxiolytic sedatives would seem to be a sensible approach to the problem. In other cases, frigidity is a reflection of social inhibitions which are frequently, it has been said, 'soluble in alcohol'.

A more specific approach to the problems of impotence and frigidity, using the techniques of behaviour therapy, has recently been devised (see chapter 8).

2 *Opiates and psychodysleptics* In the East it is still widely held that opium increases the pleasures of sexual activity, and because

of its sedative action, reduces the likelihood of premature ejaculation. While this may be true for the occasional user, it is quite clear that morphine and heroin addicts are almost completely lacking in sexual drive.

LSD has been alleged to have aphrodisiac properties but this is almost certainly illusory. Rather than producing a heightening of true sexual desires, it produces what Havelock Ellis aptly called 'an orgy of vision'.

Cannabis is also endowed with aphrodisiac properties by some and is frequently taken in Egypt to improve a waning sexuality. When taken regularly, however, it has the opposite effect: 'A Romeo who took hashish would quickly have forgotten Juliet' (*Gautier*).

3 *Psychostimulants* Amphetamines, by combating fatigue and heightening desire, can occasionally prolong sexual activity. In most cases, however, they reduce potency by their sympathomimetic action.

Androgens

We have already seen how the strength of sexual drive in both sexes is determined, at least partly, by the level of circulating androgens. Androgens do not, however, affect reduced potency unless the impotence is a reflection of impaired testicular function. They do not influence homosexual tendencies. Ageing can lead to primary testicular failure and consequent androgen deficiency: this may be more common than was previously thought.

A few cases of impotence are associated with hyperprolactinaemia. As dopamine (DA) is believed to be the neurotransmitter responsible for inhibiting prolactin secretion (see chapter 2), treatment with a centrally acting DA agonist, such as bromocriptine, would appear to be a rational approach to the problem of hyperprolactinaemic impotence. And indeed bromocriptine has been reported as having been successful in this syndrome in restoring potency. It must be remembered, however, that hyperprolactinaemic impotence is uncommon, while psychogenic impotence is common.

Androgens have been reported as helping certain cases of frigidity in women.

Drugs acting on the autonomic system

As impotence is usually due to increased sympathetic activity, direct sympathetic inhibition might improve potency. Yohimbine, an alkaloid derived from the bark of a West African tree is an adrenergic alpha-receptor blocking agent. This might be the basis of its postulated aphrodisiac qualities, although as yet there is no direct evidence of its efficacy. Propranolol, a beta-receptor blocking agent, has also been tried in psychogenic impotence, but without success. In animals, p-chlorophenylalanine, which reduces brain levels of 5HT, appears to increase total sexual activity. As yet the effects on human sexuality remain to be investigated.

Finally, thioridazine, a phenothiazine compound (see chapter 6) possesses marked anti-adrenergic properties and has been used for premature ejaculation, as has clomipramine.

Local irritants

Cantharidin is a non-volatile anhydride present in a particular species of beetle (*Cantharis vesicatoria*), popularly called 'Spanish fly'. When ingested it irritates the gastrointestinal tract and during its excretion in the urine causes irritation of the urinary tract. It is this irritative action on the lower urinary tract which is supposed to heighten sexual desire. Whether or not it is effective, cantharidin is extremely dangerous, and fatalities have been reported.

Drugs which reduce sexual drive and performance

Oestrogens

Oestrogens can effectively reduce sexual drive in men, but this may be accompanied by irreversible gynaecomastia. Their effects in women are less predictable (see below).

Anti-androgens

Recently synthetic anti-androgen compounds have been synthesised, which are non-feminising. Cyproterone has this property and is said to be useful in suppressing sexual desire. Provera is a synthetic progestogen which antagonises testosterone. It too has been claimed to reduce libido.

Psychotropic drugs

Anxiolytic sedatives and alcohol which can, if taken in too high a dosage, lead to a reduced sexual performance, have already been discussed (see chapter 8).

Phenothiazine derivatives rarely reduce potency in men, but may well affect sexual function in women. Oligomenorrhoea, impaired ovulation and failure of uterine implantation of the fertilised ovum have all been reported. As these compounds possibly act on hypothalamic centres (see chapter 6), it is not surprising that they influence pituitary function which itself is under hypothalamic control.

Antidepressants, both the dibenzazepines as well as the mono-amine oxidase inhibitors, frequently lead to partial impotence in men or to ejaculatory difficulties. It is important for the prescribing doctor to be aware of these possibilities, as interference with sexual function may well cause a patient to stop taking his psychotropic drug with consequent deterioration in his mental state.

Drugs acting on the autonomic system

Adrenergic neurone-blocking drugs, particularly guanethidine (Ismelin) and bethanidine (Esbatal), may produce impotence, but more commonly failure of ejaculation.

Psychological effects of oral contraceptives

Between a quarter and a third of all women not on oral contraceptives notice that they tend to become somewhat depressed in the two or three days preceding their menstrual period. This depression is frequently accompanied by irritability and headache and occurs at the time of the month when the levels of circulating oestrogens and progesterone reach their peak. It is known that prolonged administration of progestogens frequently leads to depressive symptoms and marked reduction in sexual drive. There have been a number of studies of the psychological effects accompanying regular monthly administration of oral contraceptive preparations containing a mixture of an oestrogenic compound with a progestogen. While some women notice a definite improvement in their mood with oral contraceptives, rather more complain of a pronounced worsening of premenstrual depression and loss of libido. These inconsistencies do not appear to be related to the exact nature of the oestrogens or progestogens used, or, within limits, to their relative concentrations, although some women seem to do better on one preparation than another.

Drug treatment of sexual problems

Impotence and frigidity

In the great majority of cases these symptoms are entirely psychogenic and may be improved by anxiolytic sedatives which should be taken some one or two hours before retiring. The appropriate dosage may take some time to determine, as too little will be ineffective while too much will cause sedation. A benzodiazepine derivative like diazepam 2–5 mg may be used. Often an alcoholic 'nightcap' is as effective.

If this relatively non-specific approach fails, specific desensitisation with methohexitone or propanidid should be tried (see chapter 8).

In those cases which are unequivocally due to pathologically low levels of circulating androgens, testosterone propionate 5–10 mg injected once or twice a week or a testosterone implant containing 100–500 mg may be useful. Those uncommon cases of hyperprolactinaemic impotence should respond to the dopamine agonist bromocriptine (Parlodel) in a dose of 5–10 mg a day.

Finally, in cases where the adrenergic neurone-blocking drug bethanidine is being taken, omission of the evening dose may lead to satisfactory sexual function.

Sexual deviations

Sexual deviation is more common among men than among women, and men are more likely to commit grave antisocial acts in order to gratify their sexual desires. While no pharmacological agent can by itself alter the direction of sexual desire, oestrogens will reduce its strength. Either stilboestrol 5–10 mg daily or ethinyl oestradiol 0·02–0·05 mg daily can be used. Common side-effects include nausea and gynaecomastia. Such an approach should only be considered when the sexual deviation is causing considerable distress to the individual concerned or there is a real danger of antisocial acts being committed. It is obvious that the wholehearted cooperation of the patient is necessary.

The anti-androgen compound, cyproterone acetate in a daily dose of 10–20 mg given under controlled conditions has been shown to reduce libido and to reduce the erectile response to erotic stimulation. This effect of cyproterone is accompanied by a reduction of plasma testosterone. The DA receptor blocking compound benperidol (Anquil) although having a slight but definite affect on libido in a dose of 1 mg daily, does not appear to affect plasma testosterone levels.

An altogether different approach to sexual deviation involves the attempt to desensitise the patient to any possible anxieties he may have regarding normal heterosexual intercourse. This is based on the belief that many sexual perversions arise because of difficulties, either real or imagined, with heterosexual intercourse; relieving these difficulties should remove the need for deviant behaviour. Considerable success for this approach has been claimed in the treatment of homosexuality, particularly when combined with other behavioural techniques like aversion therapy.

Suggestions for further reading

BANCROFT, J., 'The relationship between hormones and sexual behaviour in humans', in *Biological Determinants of Sexual Behaviour*, ed. J. Hutchinson, John Wiley, Chichester, 1977.

BEAUMONT, G., 'Untoward effects of drugs on sexuality' in *Psychosexual Problems*, ed. S. Crown, Academic Press, London, 1976.

GROUNDS, D. DAVIES, B., and MOWBRAY, R., The contraceptive pill, side, effects and personality', *British Journal of Psychiatry*, vol. 116, 1970, pp. 169–72.

HASLAM, M. T., 'Psycho-sexual disorders and their treatment', *Current Medical Research and Opinion*, vol. 3, 1976, pp. 726–35.

HERTZBERG, B., and COPPEN, A., 'Changes in psychological symptoms in women taking oral contraceptives'. *British Journal of Psychiatry*, vol. 116, 1970, pp. 161–4.

MASTERS, W. H., and JOHNSON, V. E., *Human Sexual Response*, Churchill, London, 1966.

PERRY, J. S., 'Effects of pharmacologically active substances on sexual function', *Journal of Reproduction and Fertility*, Supplement No. 4, 1968.

ROYAL COLLEGE OF GENERAL PRACTITIONERS, *Oral Contraceptives and Health*, Pitman, London, 1974.

I 3 Disorders of appetite and body weight

Regulation of food intake and body weight

In most people energy intake, in the form of food, is closely matched to the energy expended by exercise and metabolic needs; and body weight remains more or less constant. When energy intake exceeds expenditure, due either to an increased food consumption without a concomitant increase in energy expenditure, or to a reduced expenditure without a concomitant reduction in food intake, body weight will increase. In other words a positive energy balance leads to weight gain. Conversely, a negative energy balance leads to weight loss.

Many factors contribute to both sides of the energy balance equation. Food intake is determined by physiological mechanisms in the central nervous system and in the periphery (see below), by psychological cues such as the sight, smell and taste of food, by the overt desire to gain or lose weight, which itself is often largely socially determined, and by clinical conditions such as depressive illness which usually causes a profound loss of appetite and secondary reduction in food intake (see chapter 7). Drugs too can profoundly affect the desire to eat; for example, chlorpromazine frequently increases appetite and leads to a significant weight gain in patients receiving it for long-term management of chronic schizophrenia (see chapter 6); while other drugs such as amphetamine reduce appetite, and consequently lead to weight loss. To understand how such drugs might act we need to consider the physiological mechanism underlying the regulation of food intake.

Central nervous system

Until recently it was assumed, on the basis of earlier experiments on laboratory animals, that the hypothalamus held pride of place in the regulation of food intake, with the lateral hypothalamus being responsible for initiating feeding behaviour (the so-called 'feeding centre') and the ventro-medial hypothalamus being responsible for stopping eating (the so-called 'satiety centre'). It is now realised that this 'dual-centre' theory is an oversimplification. The two areas of the hypothalamus concerned contain many fibres from neurones arising in the brain stem which themselves affect feeding behaviour in animals. For example the lateral hypothalamus is closely associated anatomically with the median forebrain bundle in which there are dopaminergic (DA) pathways coming from the substantia nigra and associated structures, and noradrenergic (NA) fibres arising from the locus coeruleus and other brain stem nuclei (see Figure 1). Lesions made in the dopaminergic pathways outside the hypothalamus produce the syndrome of aphagia and adipsia which was previously thought to be characteristic only of lateral hypothalamic lesions. Furthermore neurones utilising 5-hydroxytryptamine (5HT) arising in the median raphe nuclei are also thought to be involved in feeding. In addition, other pathways descending from higher centres can influence feeding. Thus the neural regulation of food intake is now recognised to be extremely complex, and we can no longer talk of a single 'feeding centre' or 'satiety centre', each acting reciprocally on the other. It is more likely that many neuronal systems closely interact and no simple neurochemical or neuroanatomical theory can fully explain the regulation of food intake. Nevertheless the hypothalamus does play a part over and above that of acting as a simple relay station. Certain neurones in the lateral hypothalamus of the monkey have been found to respond to the sight of food only when the animal is food deprived, thus the lateral hypothalamus may act as a form of gating mechanism allowing certain stimuli to initiate feeding behaviour in one condition (food-deprivation) but not in another.

It may be that certain pathways, especially the DA pathways, are more concerned with the execution of feeding behaviour while others are responsible for triggering off the behaviour: if this were so lesions in the DA pathways would reduce food intake, not by reducing the desire to eat (i.e. hunger) but by impairing the ability of the animal to eat. The NA pathways on the other hand could be more concerned with initiating feeding through a hunger mechanism which may be linked to some sort of general reward system. Even here the situation is not straightforward, for lesions in the ventral NA system which produce a marked increase in food intake reminiscent of ventromedial hypothalmic lesions, are dependent for their effect on an intact pituitary gland; so there would appear to be endocrine interactions as well.

Peripheral mechanisms

1 *Blood sugar and insulin*   It has long been known that insulin, which sharply lowers blood sugar, leads to a pronounced increase in subjective hunger, a property which has at times been made use of in treatment (see below). Closer examination of the relationship of blood sugar and hunger has revealed that this increased hunger does not begin to be experienced until the blood sugar starts to rise. As a result it has been suggested that it is not the absolute level of blood sugar but the rate of utilisation which is important in this connection. When there is a lot of insulin available and glucose utilisation is high there is no increase in hunger; it is only when the rate of glucose utilisation falls, and there is a reduced arterio-venous glucose difference, that hunger occurs. This view, often referred to as the 'glucostatic theory' is compatable with the clinical observation that diabetic patients with high blood sugar levels but low glucose utilisation rates due to lack of insulin, and a consequently low arterio-venous glucose difference, often feel very hungry. It should be emphasised however that within the physiological range of blood sugar utilisation rates there is little relationship to hunger; it would appear that the glucostatic mechanism acts only in conditions of extreme food deprivation.

2 *Carbohydrate absorption*   The rate of absorption of carbohydrate from the gastrointestinal tract into the hepatic portal vein appears to influence feeding in animals. The monitoring of this carbohydrate absorption may take place through glucoreceptors in the liver and signalled to the brain via the vagus.

It is difficult to known how important this mechanism is in man; vagotomy for peptic ulcer is not usually followed by obvious changes in subjective hunger. On the other hand rapid transit of food into the small intestine and subsequent rapid absorption does produce a syndrome (the 'dumping' syndrome) in which anorexia is a component. In any case rapid absorption of glucose calls forth a sharp rise in insulin secretion which in turn may affect hunger either via the glucostatic mechanism discussed above, or perhaps by a direct action in the central nervous system.

3 *Gastro-intestinal motility*   Perhaps the earliest theory of hunger regulation was that of Cannon who attributed the sensation of hunger almost entirely to contractions of the empty stomach which caused so-called 'hunger pangs'. Subsequent work has tended to cast doubt on this mechanism as a dominant factor, although in certain normal subjects periods of fasting gastric motility, which occur every 40 to 120 minutes and which last for some 15–20 minutes on average, are associated with a detectable increase in hunger ratings (see chapter 4), conversely the disappearance of this gastric motility is accompanied by a fall in hunger ratings. Furthermore on direct questioning the majority of normal people recognise a gastro-intestinal component to their hunger sensations, although it is by no means certain that this is related to fasting gastric motility. An alternative view suggests that it is the rate of gastric emptying after a meal which determines the onset of hunger for the next meal. In keeping with this is the finding in experimental animals that administration of cholecystokinin (CKK), which is normally released when food enters the duodenum, can cause an animal to stop eating. In addition, phenylalanine, a potent releaser of CKK, is more satiating to monkeys than an isocaloric equivalent less likely to release CKK. Similar results have been obtained in man; phenylalanine was significantly more effective than placebo in causing an increase in satiety and a fall in hunger. Direct infusion of CKK in man has produced conflicting results; slow infusion actually increased food intake, a finding contrary to that expected, but rapid injection did decrease food intake. It remains to be determined whether the satiating activity of phenylalanine is due to release of CKK.

4 *Temperature and metabolic rate*   It has been suggested that we eat merely to keep warm. Certainly food intake increases in cold weather, and temperature regulation could therefore be a significant determinant of food intake. In western society, however, the ambient temperature indoors is usually controlled to within very narrow limits by such devices as central heating and air conditioning, and when we go out into the cold weather we simply put on extra clothing, thereby literally insulating ourselves against the more extreme temperatures. It may nevertheless be the case that temperature has a bearing on food intake in certain circumstances.

Changes in metabolic rate certainly can affect food intake. It is a frequent clinical observation that patients suffering from hyperthyroidism with a consequent increase in metabolic rate, are voraciously hungry. In fact, significant loss of weight in spite of a greatly increased food intake is almost pathognomonic of hyperthyroidism. The links between changes in metabolic rate and changes in hunger and food intake have yet to be determined.

Certain obese patients, who, it must be emphasised, form but a very small proportion of the whole population of obese subjects, have been found under carefully controlled conditions to have a lower than normal metabolic rate. Even restricting their intake to 4·4 MJ (1000 cals) per day is insufficient to produce weight loss, as their energy expenditure is even lower. It would appear that in those patients the regulating links between food intake and energy expenditure have been overcome by the social determinants of what constitutes a normal food intake, which in western society is well above 4·4 MJ per day.

The pharmacology of drugs affecting appetite

Drugs affecting appetite and food intake fall sharply into two groups:

1 Those which reduce hunger—appetite suppressants or *anorectics*
2 Those which increase hunger

Appetite suppressant drugs

These are of three main types:

1 Drugs acting primarily on the central nervous system
2 Drugs influencing carbohydrate metabolism
3 Bulk agents acting directly on the gastro-intestinal tract

1   *Centrally acting compounds*   All the preparations in this group, except mazindol, can be classified as phenylethylamine derivatives. Mazindol is an indol derivative.

(a) *Amphetamine*   This was the first anorectic compound to be introduced into clinical practice, and has been the most widely studied from the pharmacological point of view. Its anorectic action was noted as a chance finding in patients who had been prescribed the drug for narcolepsy. In fact the use of amphetamine as a stimulant in narcolepsy only came after a similar chance observation that when prescribed as a nasal decongestant (its original indication) it had a stimulant activity.

In man amphetamine has a well-documented anorectic effect and has been widely used in the treatment of obesity. Unfortunately its stimulant activity has led to misuse and the drug has largely been withdrawn for use in obesity. Nevertheless its pharmacology continues to be studied enthusiastically as it has a number of psychopharmacological properties of great interest. These include the stimulant activity already referred to, a euphoriant action, an anorectic effect and a peripheral sympathomimetic action. In addition large doses can produce a paranoid psychosis closely resembling paranoid schizophrenia (see chapter 6). Therefore examination of its mode of action within the central nervous system could well increase our understanding of the central mechanisms underlying hunger, mood, arousal and psychosis; those relating to mood and psychosis being particularly relevant to psychiatry.

It is currently believed that the central effects of amphetamine depend on its actions on the catecholamine pathways within the brain (see Figure 1).

Amphetamine, particularly the dextrorotatory (+) isomer, releases preformed NA and DA from the nerve terminals, and to a lesser extent blocks their active reuptake. There is some evidence in both man and experimental animals that the euphoriant and stimulant activity of amphetamine is mediated by DA pathways, as the effects are blocked by specific DA receptor blocking drugs such as pimozide (see chapter 6). Its anorectic action on the other hand is thought by some to be mediated by the ventral NA pathway, as destruction of this pathway in rats attenuates the anorectic effect of amphetamine. Although in man at least, dopamine receptor blockade by pimozide does not appear to influence amphetamine anorexia, the evidence on this point from animal studies is conflicting, and the question of the mode of action of amphetamine on hunger remains unresolved.

Amphetamine psychosis is more fully discussed in chapters 6 and 10, suffice it to say here that this might well be mediated via a dopamine pathway involving the limbic cortex.

The sympathomimetic activity of amphetamine gives rise to cardiovascular symptoms (palpitations), dry mouth and dilatation of the pupil.

The subject of amphetamine abuse is covered in chapter 10.

(b) *Phenmetrazine, phentermine and diethylpropion* All three of these compounds have some central stimulant activity as well as an anorectic one. This is particularly pronounced in the case of phenmetrazine which has been used, like amphetamine, as a drug of abuse. The other two drugs, phentermine and diethylpropion while showing stimulant activity under laboratory conditions, for example they both increase critical flicker frequency (see chapter 4), have not been so prone to abuse.

The central pharmacology of this group of drugs is similar to amphetamine, they appear to act on the catecholamine systems in the brain. It may be, however, that phentermine and diethylpropion have a greater relative effect on NA as compared to DA pathways, and thus have less stimulant and euphoriant activity than amphetamine for an equipotent anorectic dose. This suggestion would explain some of the differences between them. It should be pointed out that both drugs can cause an amphetamine-like psychosis although the number of reported cases of psychosis is extremely small compared to the number of prescriptions issued.

(c) *Fenfluramine* Although chemically similar to amphetamine, and although showing an anorectic activity, fenfluramine has sedative rather than stimulant properties and has been associated with a depression of mood rather than an elevation. It is thought to act primarily on the 5HT pathways rather than NA or DA. In animals the anorectic action of fenfluramine is impaired by drugs such as methysergide and cyproheptadine which block 5HT receptors and by drugs which destroy 5HT containing neurones, such as 5, 6-dihydroxytryptamine.

Not only does the neurochemical basis of fenfluramine's anorectic action differ from that of amphetamine, but its effects on the eating behaviour of rats also differs. Whereas amphetamine delays the onset of eating, fenfluramine reduces the size of the meal without affecting its onset. On the basis of such observations amphetamine has been said to act on 'hunger' and fenfluramine on 'satiety'. Whether or not this is true in man is undetermined. It is, of course, only in man that hunger and satiety can be directly explored; investigations in animals are limited to observing feeding behaviour, and it may be unwarranted to extrapolate from one to the other.

Fenfluramine has a peripheral action as well as a central one; it increases the uptake of glucose into muscle cells. This peripheral effect may play a part in its efficacy in the treatment of obesity (see below).

(d) *Mazindol* This is the most novel of the clinically available anorectic drugs and its pharmacology is not so well understood as the others. The most recent view is that it acts on both NA and DA pathways by preventing reuptake; whether or not it has a similar action on 5HT pathways is uncertain.

2 Drugs affecting carbohydrate metabolism

(a) *Glucagon* This is a hormone produced by the α cells of the pancreas which elevates blood-sugar levels and increases the a/v glucose gradient.

While glucagon does lead to a reduction in both subjective hunger and food intake in healthy subjects as would be predicted by the glucostatic theory, the maximum effect is not observed until some two hours following intramuscular injection, occuring later than the blood-sugar effect. It may be that glucagon influences some other factor, such as gastric motility, which in turn affects the hypothalamus. Measures of gastric motility have shown that glucagon does indeed reduce motility, but again the maximum reduction in motility occurs rather earlier than the maximum hunger reduction.

(b) *Biguanides* Two compounds in this group, metformin (Glucophage) and phenformin (Dibotin), which have a hypoglycaemic action, are widely used in the treatment of diabetes mellitus, particularly the maturity-onset type commonly associated with obesity. It was noticed that obese diabetic patients appeared to lose weight much more easily while they were taking metformin or phenformin than on diet alone.

The mechanism by which these compounds affect body weight is obscure. In diabetics they increase the peripheral utilisation of glucose by improving the insulin clearance in muscle as compared to adipose tissue. Yet in non-diabetic obese subjects, where there is also a reduced peripheral glucose uptake, the biguanides do not improve peripheral glucose uptake, but probably act by reducing gluconeogenesis. It is debatable whether the biguanide compounds have a true anorectic action, as distinct from producing nausea.

3 *Bulk agents* As methylcellulose was observed to swell in the presence of water it was hoped that if it were swallowed it would similarly swell inside the stomach and thereby produce a feeling of satiety. No direct evidence of any such effect has been produced. In a series of carefully controlled observations, doses of methyl-cellulose of up to 3 g (9 tablets) led to no detectable reduction of either measured food intake or subjective hunger ratings. Equally, controlled clinical trials of these substances in obese subjects have failed to reveal any significant weight reduction attributable to them.

Appetite stimulating drugs

1 *Insulin* Both exogenous insulin administration and endo-genous hypersecretion, as occurs in spontaneous hypoglycaemia, are accompanied by a marked increase in subjective hunger. From experimental studies it is clear that this hunger does not appear until the blood sugar has reached its lowest point and is beginning to rise, that is, some thirty minutes after administration. It may be of significance that the onset of hunger occurs at approximately the same time as the appearance of pronounced fasting gastric motility. However, it is likely that both the subjective awareness of hunger and the occurrence of gastric motility are themselves secondary to hypothalamic activity.

2 *Phenothiazines* Chlorpromazine (Largactil) and its deriva-tives, which are widely used in the treatment of schizophrenia (see chapter 6), frequently lead to considerable weight gain; in some series virtually all patients on continuous phenothiazine medication were noted to have gained weight, with some becoming distinctly obese. Those who develop marked adiposity report that the medication seems to make them feel voraciously hungry.

As careful studies have failed to reveal any metabolic cause for the increase in weight observed, it is likely that these compounds directly affect the hunger-regulating mechanism in the hypothala-mus. Recent experimental evidence supports this view; direct injection of chlorpromazine into the lateral hypothalamus pro-moted increased food intake in animals.

3 *Cyproheptadine (Periactin)* This compound, which has anti-histaminic properties and which also antagonises the activity of

5-hydroxytryptamine, was introduced clinically as an anti-histamine. Patients receiving it were noted to gain weight and laboratory animals were shown to consume more calories when cyproheptadine was given. In addition, significant weight gain was observed in both children and adults following cyproheptadine administration, as compared to that occurring after placebo. The assumption was made that the observed increase in weight reflected an underlying rise in hunger, and a consequent increase in food intake. Evidence has been obtained which substantiates this view; a group of young adults were shown to feel significantly more hungry when taking cyproheptadine than when taking placebo. This effect could be related to the compound's anti-5HT activity, particularly as 5HT occurs in the hypothalamus in high concentration.

Drug treatment of appetite disorders

The two clinical conditions in which disturbances of body weight and appetite are of primary importance are obesity and psychogenic malnutrition (anorexia nervosa). In obesity there is an excess of adipose tissue, arising from more calories being consumed than are expended, while psychogenic malnutrition develops if more calories are expended than are consumed. The rational treatment of each situation is to reverse the calorie imbalance which has occurred. In both situations it is the appropriate dietary regime which is of fundamental importance; the place of drugs is secondary, they should only be used as adjuncts to dietary treatment, never as a substitute for it.

Obesity

For most clinical purposes body weight will suffice as an index of the degree of adiposity present; an individual can be considered as clinically obese if he exceeds his ideal body weight by 20 per cent. When this level of overweight is reached it is time for treatment to be instituted. Treatment should be based on appropriate dietary advice, together with an admonition to take frequent, but moderate, exercise. In most cases patients will require close supervision and support which is best provided by their family doctor seeing them initially at weekly or fortnightly intervals. Such supportive care is particularly important in those patients whose obesity is a consequence of psychological disturbance. Although such patients form a minority of the overweight subjects in the population they are usually the ones who find it the most difficult to keep to a diet. Their eating pattern is not only determined by physiological requirements; psychological needs play a great part. They find that food, particularly sweet food, helps to reduce their anxiety or depression and therefore suffer greater temptations to break their diet than the majority of obese patients who have no such underlying psychological disturbance.

Appetite suppressant drugs can in some cases provide a useful addition to combined dietary and supportive treatment, but should not be used as the sole treatment.

Although amphetamine was the first centrally acting anorectic drug to be introduced, its central stimulant and euphoriant properties led to it becoming a drug of abuse (see chapter 10). Because of this most authorities now recommend that amphetamine (Benzedrine) and its dextro-isomer (Dexedrine) should not be used in the treatment of obesity; particularly as more satisfactory alternatives are now available. The same strictures apply to phenmetrazine (Preludin).

1 *Diethylpropion* (*Tenuate*, *Apisate*) While diethylpropion has an anorectic effect equal to that of amphetamine, clinically it does not appear to produce the same degree of central stimulation as amphetamine or phenmetrazine. Equally the risk of drug dependence seems to be less. Nevertheless, there is good experimental evidence to suggest that it can have a stimulant effect on the CNS as measured by CFF, and caution should therefore be applied when prescribing it.

Several controlled studies have revealed its efficacy in the treatment of obesity with daily weight losses of 20–80 g being directly attributable to the anorectic effect produced. It has shown to be the most effective when taken in doses of 50 mg one and one-half to two hours before meals. Equally effective clinically is the long-acting preparation (Tenuate dospan) which contains 75 mg diethylpropion in a slow release form.

Intermittent treatment, with alternating months on diethylpropion and placebo, has proved almost as effective as continuous treatment. As such a regime reduces the likelihood of drug dependence, it is to be preferred to continuous medication.

2 *Phentermine* Phentermine when prescribed intermittently (30 mg daily) over a period of thirty-six weeks was found to be as effective, in terms of weight loss, as continuous administration, and more effective than placebo.

3 *Fenfluramine (Ponderax)* Clinically, fenfluramine (in doses from 40–120 mg daily) is an effective adjunct to weight reduction regimes, being associated with weight losses similar to those of the other compounds previously discussed. Its main distinction from those compounds is its complete lack of any stimulant properties; if anything, it has a mild sedative action which is particularly useful in the treatment of those obese patients who also show signs of anxiety. Unfortunately it too has drawbacks, being prone to produce gastrointestinal side-effects, particularly diarrhoea, and acute confusional states following fenfluramine administration have been observed, particularly among patients who were receiving monoamine oxidase inhibitors at the same time. It is important to note that sudden withdrawal of fenfluramine can lead to overt depression. Reduction of dosage should therefore be undertaken gradually, and intermittent treatment with fenfluramine is not advised.

4 *Mazindol (Teronac, Sanorex)* This drug possesses a definite, relatively long lasting anorectic action which has proved useful in the treatment of obesity. The recommended dose is 2 mg daily given orally in the morning. Whether or not it has any advantages over diethylpropion or phentermine is uncertain, as pronounced sympathomimetic effects and some central stimulant activity have been reported.

5 *Biguanide compounds—Metformin (Glucophage) and phenformin (Dibotin)* While these compounds certainly assist obese diabetics in losing weight, their place in the treatment of uncomplicated obesity is still uncertain. At present their use should be restricted to those obese patients who are also suffering from diabetes mellitus, or who are thought to be pre-diabetic; for these patients the biguanides would appear to be the treatment of choice. The recommended doses are: metformin 0·5–1·0 g or phenformin 25–50 mg, three times daily.

6 *Bulk agents—Methylcellulose (Cellevac, Cellucon)* As there is no reliable clinical or experimental evidence to substantiate the

claim that methylcellulose reduces hunger or food intake, preparations containing methylcellulose have little place in the treatment of obesity.

7 *General recommendations* It cannot be stressed too strongly or too often that successful weight reduction can only result from reducing intake of calories to a level below that expended. All the preparations discussed above can therefore only be considered as possible adjuncts to a sensible dietary programme and never as complete treatments in themselves.

Furthermore, if an appetite-suppressant drug of the mildly stimulant type such as diethylpropion or phentermine is used it should be prescribed intermittently and not continuously; patients should be on the drug for one or two months at the most, spending a similar period without medication before it is prescribed again. With these provisos, diethylpropion or phentermine would appear the most suitable anorectic compounds for depressed, lethargic, obese patients, while fenfluramine is probably better for the anxious, overactive patient. Obese diabetics should benefit most from one of the biguanide compounds.

Anorexia nervosa (Psychogenic malnutrition)

Anorexia nervosa is a condition in which severe malnutrition occurs as a result of a deliberate attempt by the patient to lose weight, usually because of a pathological fear of being fat. This characteristically takes the form of drastic reduction in calorie intake, although self-induced vomiting or frequent purgation may also be practised.

Anorexia nervosa most often begins during adolescence or in early adult life, affecting females far more frequently than males. In girls, amenorrhoea supervenes sooner or later. Despite the name of the condition, appetite is preserved in many cases. The emaciation produced, although alarming, is completely reversible by dietary measures.

The place of drugs in this condition, if any, is to assist the patient to keep to the diet and thereby gain weight. Apart from general sedation which may be required in the case of a particularly uncooperative patient, certain drugs are considered by some to have a particular value in helping patients to gain weight; these are chlorpromazine and insulin.

1 *Chlorpromazine (Largactil)* Chlorpromazine and to a lesser degree other phenothiazine derivatives frequently increase appetite and produce weight gain in psychiatric patients requiring to take them over long periods. In addition they have a marked sedative effect. It is just this combination of hunger stimulation and sedation which is particularly suitable for anorexia nervosa. In many patients, however, no such medication is required as they readily settle in hospital and regain their appetite spontaneously, if they ever lose it. For those who do not respond to such relatively simple measures, chlorpromazine can usefully be prescribed in doses from 100 mg three times daily, increasing to the level of tolerance. Care must be taken to avoid over-sedation, and the occurrence of parkinsonian symptoms will require appropriate anti-parkinsonian medication, together with a reduction in dosage of chlorpromazine.

A complication observed in some 10 per cent of the patients receiving chlorpromazine for anorexia nervosa is grand mal epilepsy.

2 *Insulin* As we have seen, subcutaneous injection of insulin leads to an increase in hunger some thirty minutes later. It is therefore not surprising that insulin has long been used to encourage patients with anorexia nervosa to eat, but obviously this measure will only be of value in those patients who are truly anorectic. The usual practice is to begin by injecting 10 units of soluble insulin one hour after breakfast. The dosage is then increased each day until sweating and slight drowsiness is produced; when these effects are observed a meal is offered to the patient, which, if eaten, will counter them. In general 40–60 units prove sufficient for the purpose. Patients receiving this treatment must be closely observed for several hours after the injection and a 20-ml-syringe containing a solution of glucose suitable for intravenous administration must be kept readily available in case sudden profound hypoglycaemia occurs.

3 *Cyproheptadine* (Periactin) A controlled trial of cyproheptadine in anorexia nervosa has revealed that it is probably of some benefit in the treatment of anorexia nervosa, particularly where this is undertaken under out-patient conditions.

Suggestions for further reading

Regulation of food intake

BALAGURA, S., *Hunger*, Basic Books, New York, 1973.

BLUNDELL, J. E., 'Is there a role for serotonin in feeding ?', *International Journal of Obesity*, vol. 1, 1977, pp. 15–42.

NOVIN, D., WYRWICKA, W., and BRAY, G., *Hunger: Basic Mechanisms and Clinical Implications*, Raven Press, New York, 1976.

SILVERSTONE, T., ed., *Appetite and Food Intake*, Dahlem Konferenzen, Berlin, 1976.

Pharmacology of drugs affecting appetite

GARATTINI, S., BIZZI, G., DE GAENTANO, A., JORI, A., and SAMANIN, S., 'Recent advances in the pharmacology of anorectic agents', in *Recent Advances in Obesity Research*, ed. A. Howard, Newman Publishing, London, 1975.

GARATTINI, S., and SAMANIN, T., 'Anorectic drugs and brain neuro-transmitters', in *Appetite and Food Intake*, ed. T. Silverstone, Dahlem Konferenzen, Berlin, 1976.

KIRBY, M. J., and TURNER, P., 'Do "anorectic" drugs produce weight loss by appetite suppression ?', *Lancet*, vol. 1, 1976, pp. 566–7.

PAYKEL, E. S., MUELLER, P. S., and DE LA VERGNE, P. M., 'Amitriptyline weight gain and carbohydrate craving', *British Journal of Psychiatry*, vol. 123, 1973, pp. 501–7.

ROBINSON, R. G., MCHUGH, P. R., and FOLSTEIN, M. F., 'Measurement of appetite disturbances in psychiatric disorders', *Journal of Psychiatric Research*, vol. 12, 1975, pp. 59–68.

SILVERSTONE, T., 'Anorectic drugs', in *Obesity: Pathogenesis and Management*, ed. T. Silverstone, Medical and Technical Publishing, Lancaster, 1975.

Disorders of appetite and body weight

BRAY, G. A., *Obesity in Perspective*, US Government Printing Office, 1975.

BRAY, G. A., *The Obese Patient*, Saunders, Philadelphia, 1976.

BRUCH, H., *Eating Disorders*, Basic Books, New York, 1974.

CRADDOCK, D., *Obesity and Its Management*, 2nd edn, Churchill Livingstone, Edinburgh, 1973.

DALLY, P., *Anorexia Nervosa*, Heinemann Medical Books, London, 1969.

GARROW, J., *Energy Balance and Obesity in Man*, North Holland, Amsterdam, 1974.

HOWARD, A., *Recent Advances in Obesity Research*, Newman Publishing, London, 1975.

JAMES, W. P. T., *Research on Obesity*, A Report of the DHSS/MRC Group, HMSO, London, 1976.

SILVERSTONE, T., *Obesity: Pathogenesis and Management*, Medical and Technical Publishing, Lancaster, 1975.

Pain

Psychophysiology of pain

Pain is more than a modality of sensation like vision, hearing or touch; it is the integrated behavioural response of an individual to a noxious stimulus, either real or imagined. The experience of pain response depends not only on the intensity of the stimulus, but also on its central interpretation. As Merskey puts it 'pain is a psychological experience of events, occurring within the patient's own body, which is always unpleasant and associated with the impression of damage to the tissues'. Pain is by no means restricted to patients with organic disease; on the contrary a considerable proportion (about 60 per cent) of patients subsequently labelled 'psychiatric' present with symptoms of pain to their general practitioners. In general medical clinics of hospitals some 40 per cent of the patients, in whom the condition is considered to be primarily a psychiatric one, complain of pain. Such non-organic pain is commonly located in the head or trunk and has an arbitrary time course, unrelated to such events as eating, posture or exercise.

Even obviously organically determined pain can be greatly affected by psychological factors. For instance in 1943 Beecher noted at Anzio that soldiers with severe war wounds complained more about clumsy venepunctures than of their lacerations. Furthermore, their analgesic requirements were often small when compared with those for more trivial injuries away from the immediate stress of battle. Another example of the close relationship between the appreciation of pain and other psychological functions is provided in the case of neuroleptanalgesia; in this technique, potent narcotic and tranquillising drugs produce changes in a patient's interpretation of stimuli, so that major surgical procedures may be carried out in the conscious state without a painful response, even though local or general anaesthetic agents have not been given.

Such observations cast serious doubt on the *specificity theory* of pain sensation which was accepted for more than a century by eminent neurologists, such as Charles Bell, Weber, Brown-Sequard and von Frey. According to this theory pain is a specific modality like vision and hearing, and possesses its own peripheral and central apparatus. The peripheral component was thought to involve the free nerve endings in the dermis. Sir Henry Head distinguished between two types of pain, one sharp (epicritic) and the other dull (protopathic), and later investigators suggested that these were mediated by nerve fibres of different size and conduction velocities. There were important drawbacks to this theory, however, and a *pattern theory* was put forward by Goldschneider, in which he postulated that the appreciation of pain depended upon both the stimulus intensity and on central summation of the afferent impulses. These two viewpoints have been linked by Melzack and Wall, into the *gate-control theory*.

Gate-control theory of pain

It is known that stimulation of the skin evokes nerve impulses that are transmitted to three systems of nerves in the spinal cord:

(i) the cells of the substantia gelatinosa in the dorsal horn of the cord
(ii) the fibres in the dorsal column that run upwards towards the brain
(iii) the first central transmission cells (T) in the dorsal horn.

Melzack and Wall proposed that the cells of the substantia gelatinosa function as a 'gate' which regulates transmission from the peripheral fibres from the skin to the T cells. The patterns of activity in the ascending neurones of the dorsal column regulate central brain processes which in turn influence the 'gate-control' activity of the cells of the substantia gelatinosa through descending fibres. Finally, the T cells activate the neural mechanisms responsible for response and perception. In other words, the cells of the substantia gelatinosa regulate the level of stimulation by impulses from the periphery of the T cells (which are the first stage of the central pain response and perception system). The amount of stimulation which these 'gate' cells permit is dependent on inhibitory and excitatory activity in large and small fibres respectively from the periphery, and on inhibition and excitation through descending pathways from the brain (see Figure 7).

This theory not only reconciles the specificity and pattern theories of pain perception, but is also consistent with other phenomena concerned with pain. For example, the intense pain associated with some forms of peripheral neuropathy, such as that due to diabetes or alcoholism, may be explained by a reduction in the normal inhibition of input by the gate-control system, because of selective large fibre destruction in these conditions.

It is probable that gating and selection of sensory information takes place at many levels of the central nervous system and that centrally acting drugs may influence this activity at various levels, so producing varying degrees and types of alteration in pain perception and response.

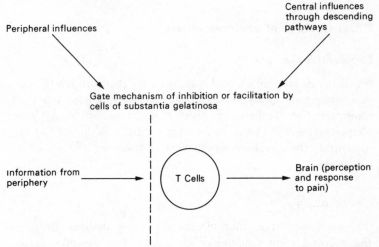

Figure 7 *Diagram to illustrate role of substantia gelatinosa in acting as a gate-control system in regulating input of sensory information into the central nervous pathways concerned with the perception of, and response to, pain*

Nature of nociceptors

Although pain may be produced by many different forms of tissue injury, it is possible that the actual stimulus common to all is chemical. A wide variety of substances produce pain when applied to exposed dermis; these include acids, alkaloids, hypo- and hypertonic solutions, histamine, 5-hydroxytryptamine, acetylcholine

231

and several polypeptides including bradykinin, angiotensin and vasopressin and prostaglandins, long-chain unsaturated fatty acid derivatives of prostanoic acid. It is likely that physical forms of injury produce their painful effects by releasing similar substances in the tissues, and it is probable that 'pain receptor' itself is chemical in nature. The term 'chemoceptor' has been coined to apply to such a receptor, which is unlikely to have a specific chemical structure, as there is such a large variety of pain-producing agents. Furthermore, it is possible that other compounds, by attaching themselves to chemoceptors, might prevent pain-producing substances from approaching the receptors sufficiently closely for binding, thus preventing the painful response. There is experimental evidence to suggest that the antipyretic analgesics act in this way.

Pharmacology of analgesic drugs

Peripheral action

Experiments in animals and man indicate that antipyretic analgesic drugs such as aspirin and paracetamol act, at least in part, by inhibiting the synthesis of prostaglandins or by blocking the chemoreceptors for pain. In keeping with this is the relative lack of central actions of these drugs when compared with the narcotic analgesics.

Central action

The most important group of centrally acting analgesic drugs are the narcotic compounds derived from the opium alkaloids, or structurally related to them. These include the potent analgesics morphine and diamorphine, and the weaker dihydrocodeine and codeine. They all possess other central effects, including sedation and respiratory depression. The narcotic antagonist compounds pentazocine and cyclazocine, which antagonise the sedation and respiratory depressant activity of the narcotic analgesic, also possess some analgesic activity which is significantly less than that of the narcotic analgesics, but may, nevertheless, be of therapeutic value. Pentazocine, in particular, has become widely used, but although its dependence-producing properties are much lower than morphine, dependence to it has been described in a few cases, and central effects of dysphoria and hallucinations are not uncommon.

The actual site and mode of action of these compounds is not known for certain, but specific brain receptors have recently been identified which possess a high affinity for morphine and morphine-like alkaloids. A small peptide with the same structures as residues 61–65 of the lipotropin chain, and with morphine-like activity in various pharmacological assays, has been identified in pig brain, and called methionine enkephalin. Another peptide, called the C-fragment consisting of residues 61–91 of lipotropin, has even greater opiate affinity than methionine enkephalin, and produces profound analgesia in the cat after intraventricular or intravenous administration. These important findings will almost certainly lead to new developments in the field of analgesic drugs.

The narcotic analgesic drugs can all produce severe disturbances of perception, leading at times to hallucinations, if given in large doses. Bradley has suggested that these analgesic and hallucinogenic actions are closely interrelated in their basic pharmacological mechanism, analgesia being a form of disturbance of sensory function similar to that which occurs in drug-induced hallucinations. In favour of this notion is the finding that the potent hallucinogen lysergic acid diethylamide (LSD) has been shown to interfere with the flow of sensory information to the cerebral cortex in animals.

Although not of therapeutic analgesic importance when used alone, some other centrally acting drugs can be shown to raise the pain threshold in animals and man. Among these are amphetamine, a central stimulant drug, and chlorpromazine, a central depressant compound. Once again, the mechanism of their analgesic effects is unknown.

Interactions of analgesic drugs

Although certain phenothiazines have an antanalgesic action in respect to experimentally induced deep somatic pain, in clinical practice most phenothiazines potentiate the effects of narcotic analgesic drugs. The phenothiazines, particularly those which are dimethylaminopropyl derivatives, are thought to act primarily by modifying entry of information into the reticular formation of the brain stem, and it is probable that their interaction with analgesic compounds is dependent on this. At the same time they help to reduce anxiety associated with the presence of severe pain, especially when this is due to malignancy.

Neuroleptanalgesia is a term given to the state of analgesia obtained by the combination of a neuroleptic agent and an analgesic of short duration. The neuroleptics most commonly used for this purpose are phenothiazines or phenothiazine derivatives, such as chlorprothixine, and butyrophenones such as droperidol. The analgesics are essentially of the morphine type: moramide, phenoperidine and phentanyl. The two types of drugs are usually given by continuous intravenous infusion. Although the patient so treated has a tendency to sleep, he need not do so, but is not particularly provoked by traumatic procedures such as surgical operation, which would normally be intolerably painful to him, thus producing a clinical state of shock. An essential part of the phenomenon is the protection of the patient against the autonomic effects of pain by selectively blocking the various cellular, autonomic and endocrine mechanisms normally active during stress. The patient is usually conscious, but not capable of prolonged attention. The corneal reflex is present, and the skin is pink, warm and dry; there is muscular hypotension and relaxation, while the respiratory rate is low and the volume increased; arterial pressure and heart rate is reduced, but tissue perfusion remains satisfactory as cardiac output increases with an associated diuresis. Body temperature usually falls, particularly when chlorprothixine is used. After recovery the patient is calm, without nausea or vomiting and remains amnesic for the procedure.

Neuroleptanalgesia emphasises the importance of central nervous factors in mediating the normal pain responses to noxious stimuli, and the way in which modification of central function may influence the nature of these responses, both physiological and autonomic.

Clinical aspects

The choice of analgesic drug for a particular patient depends on several factors:

1 *The nature of the pain-producing pathology* When pain is associated with malignancy or myocardial infarction, sedation, as well as analgesia, is required. In such circumstances the narcotic analgesic compounds with their central sedating action are to be

preferred to peripherally acting compounds. Such considerations also occur frequently after surgical procedures. In the case of non-malignant conditions, however, the number of doses should be limited to the minimum necessary to relieve pain, in order to reduce the risk of development of dependence. Pain associated with inflammatory conditions, particularly the musculoskeletal system, is better treated with antipyretic-analgesic compounds having a peripheral action.

2   *The severity of the pain*   It is a therapeutic maxim that the mildest analgesic compound should be used which produces adequate pain relief. When a peripherally acting compound is required, therefore, paracetamol and aspirin should be used before the more potent, but potentially more dangerous, compounds such as phenylbutazone (Butazolidin) and indomethacin (Indocid). Similarly, codeine and dihydrocodeine have markedly less central depressant, hallucinogenic and dependence-producing activity than the more potent compounds such as pethidine, morphine and diamorphine. Pentazocine (Fortral), a narcotic antagonist, is a weaker analgesic than morphine, but its dependence-producing properties are also less.

If a potent narcotic analgesic drug is used for only slight pain, its side-effects may more than outweigh its therapeutic advantages. In controlled clinical trials in post-operative pain, pethidine 100 mg has been found to be not significantly different from placebo when all the patients were considered overall, but if they were subdivided according to initial severity of their pain, then the drug was found to be very effective in those with severe pain, but of no value in those with only slight pain. Conversely, aspirin 600 mg was of no demonstrable value in the patient population taken overall, but was very effective in the patients with mild pain, and of little or no value in those with severe pain. This difference probably reflects the greater weight patients attach to side-effects if their pain is only slight, or if the analgesic drug is producing inadequate pain relief.

The severity of pain after any operative procedure varies greatly from patient to patient, and the practice of routine prescription of regular potent narcotic analgesic drugs for all patients after surgical operations should be discouraged. Treatment should only be prescribed after full consideration of individual requirements, even though this may take up more of the doctor's time.

3 *Other treatment which the patient is receiving* The analgesic activity of the narcotic drugs, in particular, is increased by neuroleptic drugs of the phenothiazine and butyrophenone type. For this reason smaller doses than normal of the analgesic drug may be required in patients already receiving one of the neuroleptics. Similarly, where a patient is becoming tolerant to the analgesic activity of a drug, its effectiveness may be increased by the addition of a neuroleptic to the treatment regime. This has the added advantage of reducing still further any anxiety component which may be present.

Monoamine oxidase inhibitors (see chapter 7) can also interact with narcotic analgesics, particularly pethidine, to produce profound depression of central nervous function. Various disturbances may occur such as excitation, rigidity, coma, changes in blood pressure, shock and hyperpyrexia. The basic biochemical mechanism of this interaction and its manifestations is uncertain. It is of great importance that patients receiving treatment with MAO inhibitors and who require surgical procedures should only be given pethidine with considerable caution.

4 *The psychology of the patient* The evaluation of drugs in the relief of pain is difficult, and some well controlled trials have failed to show that drugs as potent as morphine are much superior to the weaker compounds, or even a placebo (see chapter 5).

When there are grounds for feeling that a patient may be abnormally suggestible, then it may be justified to present a very weak or even inactive preparation as a preliminary therapeutic trial. If he or she responds, then the risks of serious side-effects are proportionally lower than with an active drug, even though placebo-induced side-effects are frequently described by such patients.

As we have seen, pain may be largely, if not entirely, psychologically determined in many cases. Merskey and Spear have classified the situations in which this can occur as follows: (i) psychological factors (particularly anxiety or depression) which initiate or exacerbate local physical disturbances (ii) hysterical conversion syndromes (iii) delusions or hallucinations occurring as part of a major psychiatric illness, either affective or schizophrenic.

In the first group where anxiety exacerbates the situation, an anxiolytic sedative (see chapter 8), or an antidepressant (see chapter 7), where the pain is a feature of an underlying depressive illness, will often by themselves be sufficient to relieve the pain. Muscular pains of the tension type are common in anxiety states and pain is a frequent feature of depressive illness. In the latter condition the pain may be a recurrence of past organically determined pain, or it may represent a preoccupation with bodily sensations which are normally well tolerated when the patient is well.

Pain occurring as a manifestation of conversion hysteria requires specialist psychiatric treatment. Anxiolytic sedatives and anti-depressants are unlikely to help, while the narcotic analgesics should not be given, because of the serious risk of producing drug dependency (Eugene O'Neill's play, *A Long Day's Journey into Night* provides a grim example of this).

If pain occurs as a feature of either a delusion or a hallucinatory experience the appropriate action is treatment of the psychosis (see chapter 6 for treatment of schizophrenia and chapter 7 for treatment of affective disorders).

Suggestions for further reading

ARMSTRONG, D., 'Pharmacology of pain', *British Journal of Hospital Medicine*, vol. 10, 1973, pp. 761–71.

BRADBURY, A. F., SMYTH, D. G., and SNELL, F. R., 'The peptide hormones: molecular and cellular aspects', *Ciba Foundation Symposium No. 41*, London, 1976.

BRADBURY, A. F., SMYTH, D. G., SNELL, F. R., BIRDSALL, N. J. M., and HULME, E. C., 'C fragment of lipotropin has a high affinity for brain opiate receptors', *Nature*, vol. 260, 1976, pp. 793–5.

HORN, A. S., and RODGERS, J. R., 'Structural and conformational relation-ships between the enkephalins and the opiates', *Nature*, vol. 260, 1976, pp. 795–7.

KOSTERLITZ, H. W., and HUGHES, J., 'Peptides with a morphine-like action in the brain', *British Journal of Psychiatry*, vol. 130, 1977, pp. 298–304.

LANCET (Editorial), 'Searching for the endogenous analgesic', *Lancet*, vol. 2, 1976, p. 665.

MERSKY, H., and HESTER, R. A., 'The treatment of chronic pain with psychotropic drugs', *Postgraduate Medical Journal*, vol. 48, 1972, pp. 594–8.

In general, drug treatment has but a limited place in child psychiatry. The majority of cases presenting to the child psychiatrist require social and psychotherapeutic support rather than pharmacological intervention. Nevertheless, there are certain syndromes which do benefit from psychotropic drugs. In general such drugs act through the control of a symptom rather than in producing any basic modification of the underlying disorder. Although there is some disagreement among child psychiatrists concerning the efficacy of drug treatment in the disorders which they treat, drugs have been used successfully in the following conditions: behaviour disturbance in brain damaged and epileptic children; school refusal; nocturnal enuresis; some cases of stammering; certain patients with motor tics. Those very rare cases of true schizophrenia which occur during the later stages of childhood respond to neuroleptic drugs in a similar fashion to adults (see chapter 6).

Behaviour disturbance in brain-damaged children

It is now generally recognised that psychiatric disorder is common among children showing evidence of brain damage, the most frequent abnormality being antisocial behaviour. Other syndromes thought to be a reflection of underlying cerebral pathology include the hyperkinetic syndrome, aggressive outbursts and autistic behaviour. Many brain-damaged children also suffer from epilepsy and, where this occurs, adequate control of epileptic attacks will often improve the situation considerably. Control may be achieved by phenytoin (Epanutin) 60–200 mg daily, primidone (Mysoline) 100–500 mg daily, carbamazepine (Tegretol) 100–500 mg daily, sulthiame (Ospolot) 60–300 mg daily. In addition the latter compound has been reported to improve behaviour in disturbed mentally handicapped patients who are not epileptic. As pheno-barbitone tends to exacerbate behaviour disorders it should be avoided where possible in the management of epileptic children who manifest disturbed behaviour.

In addition to epilepsy there may be other associated neuro-logical abnormalities which further complicate the life of the brain-damaged child. Thus the management of behaviour disturb-ance in children with brain damage encompasses rather more than just the prescription of an appropriate drug; a comprehensive social, psychological and physical approach is required. In fact one leading authority has gone so far as to state: 'The advice to those about to prescribe for the mentally handicapped is—when in doubt don't.' Drugs, when used for mentally handicapped patients, should be prescribed on the same basis as for children without such problems, and should in general be given for relatively brief periods only. If more prolonged treatment is required then repeated reassessments of the need for the drug should be made.

Hyperkinetic syndrome

The hyperkinetic syndrome (which is thought to be a reflection of underlying brain damage) is characterised by extreme restless-ness and distractability, usually coming on between the ages of two and five. There may or may not be frank neurological signs. Epilepsy, which complicates the picture in almost half the cases, should be controlled with a suitable anticonvulsant (see above).

Symptomatic benefit can often be obtained with a neuroleptic drug (see chapter 5), the most widely used being chlorpromazine (Largactil, Thorazine) 10–25 mg three times daily. Alternatively, haloperidol (Serenace, Haldol) can be administered unobtrusively as drops added to food in a dose of 0·05 mg/kg per day.

Paradoxically, dexamphetamine (Dexedrine), which has an arousing effect in adults, has a calmative effect on hyperkinetic activity in children; an appropriate dose is 5–10 mg daily; this may be increased to a maximum of 40 mg. Methylphenidate (Ritalin) 10–60 mg daily is an equally effective alternative. However, follow up studies have failed to reveal any advantages, in terms of emo-tional adjustment, delinquent behaviour, or academic performance, among hyperkinetic children treated with methylphenidate as compared to children not so treated. Furthermore these drugs do have some serious potential disadvantages. First, the side-effects of insomnia, tachycardia and anorexia may prove troublesome, although the insomnia can be reduced by giving the drug early in the day. Second, and of even greater potential danger, is the definite risk of producing drug dependence in later years. It has been reported that the incidence of drug abuse is higher among those children with the hyperkinetic syndrome who have received amphetamine in the past. Thus administration of these drugs should be strictly limited to those children with unequivocal symptoms and signs of the condition. Even among these there is a very good chance that considerable improvement will occur by adolescence It is therefore recommended that when amphetamines are prescribed, they should be stopped from time to time to see if they are still required.

Aggressive outbursts

The behaviour of brain-damaged children may be punctuated by short-lived outbursts of extreme aggression and destructiveness. These episodic symptoms can be ameliorated by neuroleptic drugs of the phenothiazine type (e.g. chlorpromazine) or the butyrophenone type (e.g. haloperidol). It is recommended that the use of such drugs should be limited as far as possible to controlling the outburst when it happens. A relatively uncommon condition, Gilles de la Tourette's syndrome, in which an attack of severe motor tics is accompanied by a stream of obscenities, is said to respond best to haloperidol.

School refusal and panic attacks

The extreme reluctance to go to school displayed by some children is not so much a phobia of school itself, but rather a fear of leaving the security of the home. It must be distinguished from other causes of non-attendance at school, particular truancy, which is a reflection of an antisocial attitude rather than of anxiety. Some authorities have suggested that the symptoms of school phobia can reflect underlying depression, which may be accompanied by such somatic symptoms as abdominal pain or headaches.

Although the majority of school refusers can be handled successfully without recourse to drugs, in some cases, particularly when there have been panic attacks, an anxiolytic sedative of the benzodiazepine type (see chapter 8) can reduce anxiety sufficiently to allow the child to contemplate going back to school. Chlordiazepoxide (Librium) 5–10 mg two or three times daily and diazepam (Valium) 2–5 mg three times daily are both suitable for this purpose. When used for this purpose the administration of benzodiazepines should be restricted to periods of crises, rather than given continuously. As some of these children may be depressed, the administration of an antidepressant drug of the monoamine reuptake inhibiting type (MARI), such as amitriptyline 10 to 25 mg, given as a single bed-time dose may be of value.

Nocturnal enuresis

Nocturnal enuresis, or bedwetting at night, can be considered abnormal if it persists after the age of five. It is now generally believed to be the result of delayed maturation, rather than secondary to emotional problems. In favour of this view is the observation that almost all enuretic children become completely dry at night by the time they leave school. As an approximation, some 15 per cent of children aged five frequently wet the bed at night; this figure falls to 5 per cent among 10-year-olds, and to 1 per cent by the age of 15. Rarely, nocturnal enuresis is a symptom of structural abnormality of the urinary tract, and in those cases there is usually incontinence by day as well as by night.

If physical examination and urinanalysis fail to reveal any abnormality, and the sole symptom is bedwetting, the condition is almost certainly primary nocturnal enuresis, and further investigation is rarely called for.

Drug treatment appears to help some children affected by this problem, although as yet no drug has been nearly as effective as conditioning treatment. This may take one of two forms, the first being the reinforcement of dry behaviour through the provision of a reward, normally approbation coupled with stars. The second type is required in the more severe cases; this involves the use of a bell and pad to continue the conditioning. Drugs, being so much easier to administer, are often used in the first instance in spite of the disadvantages of serious side effects and potential toxicity.

Three groups of compounds have been used: anticholinergic drugs, stimulants and tricyclic antidepressants.

Anticholinergic drugs

These act by blocking the parasympathetic innervation to the bladder. By decreasing bladder irritability and increasing urethral resistance and bladder capacity they delay bladder emptying. A wide variety of preparations have been tried, including the belladonna alkaloids, and synthetic compounds such as methantheline (Banthine) 15 mg at night, propantheline (Pro-Banthine) 15 mg at night, and isopropamide (Tyrimide) 5 mg at night. The results of treatment with these anticholinergic drugs have been generally disappointing, and frequently complicated by side effects such as dry mouth, and difficulty in visual accommodation which in turn can lead to problems with reading.

Sympathomimetic compounds

Substances such as dexamphetamine sulphate (Dexedrine), methylamphetamine (Methedrine) 5–10 mg and ephedrine 60 mg given before retiring have a dual action which would appear to be of potential benefit to enuretic subjects. They act centrally to raise cerebral arousal and should thereby lessen the depth of sleep, allowing the subject to awaken more easily when his bladder fills. They also act on the sympathetic innervation to the bladder, causing contraction of the vesical sphincter. Whatever their theoretical advantages, these drugs are of only occasional benefit in practice, and double-blind trials have not revealed any clear-cut superiority over placebo.

Tricyclic antidepressant compounds

Probably by virtue of their associated anticholinergic effects together with their known potentiation of adrenergic activity (see chapter 2), tricyclic antidepressant drugs, such as imipramine (Tofranil), amitriptyline (Tryptizol, Elavil) and nortriptyline (Aventyl), in a dose of 25–50 mg at night, have been shown to be of greater effectiveness than placebo in reducing the frequency of bedwetting. Although this is of some benefit, they only achieve the complete remission which most patients (and their parents) seek in 20 per cent of cases. Nevertheless, treatment with one of these preparations would seem to be a reasonable first step in management. If successful within three or four weeks then medication should be continued for at least another month before being cautiously reduced over the ensuing few months. Relapse during this time calls for raising the dose to the level at which a favourable response had been achieved.

If tricyclic drugs in adequate dosage fail to produce an adequate improvement within four weeks there is little point in persevering with this line of treatment, particularly as cases of tricyclic poisoning are increasing among children.

Stuttering (Stammering)

Frequent interruption of the free flow of speech, severe enough to interfere with communication, which is made worse by conscious efforts to overcome it, characterises the condition of stuttering. While this may occur to some degree in up to 3 per cent of children, only 1 per cent become persistent stutterers. As far as drug treatment is concerned, haloperidol 0·75–1·5 mg three times a day (when combined with speech therapy) has been shown to be better than a placebo given under the same conditions. Behavioural techniques which train the child to speak in a strict rhythm (by using a metronome) are also of value. Combinations of drugs with such behaviour therapy have yet to be evaluated.

Tics

Tics may be defined as brief, jerky involuntary movements, which occur particularly in the muscles around the eyes and lower part of the face. They are relatively common, being present in up to 5 per cent of all children at some time; the time they are most likely to occur is between the ages of five and ten. Tics are usually exacerbated by emotional distress, and are more frequently found in boys. Drugs of the anxiolytic sedative type such as the benzodiazepines (e.g. chlordiazepoxide 5–10 mg or diazepam 2–5 mg three times daily) may help reduce the emotional component of the condition and thereby reduce the frequency of the tics. Haloperidol 0·5–1·5 mg three times daily has also been found to be of benefit, although the larger dose may lead to extrapyramidal effects.

Sleeplessness and food refusal

These two symptoms are frequent manifestations of behaviour disturbance in early childhood. Symptomatic treatment with chlorpromazine, taken as a single 50 to 100 mg dose at night, can frequently provide sufficient control of the condition to allow any necessary environmental and attitudinal changes to take place within the family. While it is important to give an effective sedative dose, side effects, particularly a light sensitive rash, can occur. As before, drug treatment should be of limited duration being viewed merely as a way of intervening in what has become a vicious circle of interaction between parent and child.

Anorexia nervosa

See chapter 13.

Suggestions for further reading

BAIN, D. J. G., 'Prescribing psychotropic drugs for children', *Journal of the Royal College of General Practitioners*, vol. 25, 1975, pp. 49–53.

BARKER, P., *Basic Child Psychiatry*, Staples Press, London, 1971.

BARKLEY, R. A., 'A review of stimulant drug research with hyperactive children', *Journal of Child Psychology and Psychiatry*, vol. 18, 1977, pp. 137–65.

BLACKWELL, B., and CURRAN, J., 'The psychopharmacology of nocturnal enuresis', *Little Club Clinics in Developmental Medicine*, 1973.

BRITISH MEDICAL JOURNAL, editorial, 'Drugs for mentally handicapped children', vol. 1, 1976, pp. 923–4.

DRUG AND THERAPEUTICS BULLETIN, 'The management of childhood enuresis', vol. 15, 1977, pp. 26–8.

FISH, B., 'Drug use in psychiatric disorders of children', *American Journal of Psychiatry*, vol. 124, 1968, pp. 31–6.

FROMMER, E. A., 'Depressive illness in childhood', in *Affective Disorders*, ed. A. Coppen and A. Walk, *British Journal of Psychiatry*, Special Publication, no. 2., 1968.

SHAFFER, D., 'The association between enuresis and emotional disorder', *Clinics in Development Medicine*, vol. 48, 1973, p. 133.

WEISS, G., 'Effect of long term treatment of hyperactive children with methylphenidate', *Canadian Medical Association Journal*, vol. 112, 1975, pp. 159–65.

The management of overdosage of centrally acting drugs 16

Self-poisoning with centrally acting drugs, particularly barbiturates and other hypnotics, is the commonest method of suicide in the United Kingdom. There are certain general principles which apply to the treatment of such self-poisoning, irrespective of the actual substance ingested.

Maintenance of respiration

Respiratory depression occurs with many centrally acting drugs, particularly the barbiturates and other hypnotics. In addition, there may be airway obstruction due to inhalation of vomitus or to excessive mucous production. It is, therefore, of the utmost importance to ensure a clear airway, if necessary by insertion of a cuffed endotracheal tube or even by tracheostomy. If the patient is cyanosed, or in fact if there is any suspicion of inadequate ventilation, oxygen should be administered in high concentration, and intermittent positive pressure respiration considered. If facilities are available the minute volume may be measured with a Wright's spirometer and arterial blood gas analysis carried out at regular intervals. There is no place for the use of analeptic drugs in overdosage with psychotropic drugs. They have a narrow therapeutic ratio and readily produce epileptiform convulsions and cardiac dysrhythmias.

Maintenance of cardiovascular function

Depression of the vasomotor and cardiac centres may occur with many centrally acting drugs. In addition, prolonged vomiting or excessive sweating can cause marked fluid depletion and lead to a state of hypotension and shock. This results in increased sympathetic activity with peripheral vasoconstriction and shunting of blood from skin and splanchnic areas to maintain adequate coronary and cerebral perfusion. Inadequate perfusion of the lungs may lead to metabolic acidosis.

The central venous pressure should be measured and if it is reduced, intravenous fluids should be infused cautiously to increase the circulating volume and cardiac output. However, if there is any suggestion of incipient renal failure with acute tubular necrosis (see below) infusion should be delayed; equally it must be discontinued if signs of fluid excess appear. The use of vasoconstrictor agents such as noradrenaline or metaraminol is controversial. On theoretical grounds it is unlikely be of much value because sympathetic tone is already high in most shocked patients and the administration of alpha-receptor stimulating drugs may well further decrease tissue perfusion in organs such as the gut and kidney. If rehydration fails to raise the blood pressure to acceptable levels, intravenous hydrocortisone 100 mg should be given and repeated at regular intervals as necessary. Many psychotropic drugs produce cardiac dysrhythmias and cardiac monitoring should, therefore, be employed where possible during the recovery period in all patients. This is particularly true for the monoamine reuptake inhibitor antidepressant drugs, where both their anticholinergic and catecholamine reuptake inhibiting properties may play a part in production of rhythm irregularities. Anticholinesterase drugs such as intravenous physostigmine may antagonise the anticholinergic effects, and beta adrenoceptor blocking drugs such as propranolol the effects of circulating or neuronally-released catecholamines. However, they should only be regarded as adjuncts to treatment with membrane-stabilising antidysrhythmic drugs such as lignocaine administered intravenously or intramuscularly.

Control of convulsions

Convulsions may occur in overdosage with central stimulant and antidepressant compounds, and also in phenothiazine and 'Mandrax' poisoning in which the epileptic seizure threshold is reduced. They can be controlled by intramuscular injection of phenobarbitone sodium 300 mg, phenytoin sodium 250 mg, diazepam 10 mgs or paraldehyde 10 ml, repeated as necessary. If severe respiratory depression occurs, mechanical ventilation should be used.

Reduction of absorption

When it is known that the drug concerned has been ingested within four hours of admission to hospital, it is reasonable to attempt to prevent further absorption by emptying the patient's stomach or by administering activated charcoal which is said to adsorb drugs on to its surface. If the patient is conscious it may be possible to induce emesis by pharyngeal stimulation or administration of strong salt solution. The alternative for the unconscious or semi-conscious patient is gastric lavage, but this is a potentially danger-ous procedure, and must be avoided if there is any suspicion that the patient may have taken corrosives or petroleum substances, and in patients known to have upper alimentary disease. After gastric lavage has been carried out, purgation may be induced by means of 50–100 ml of 70 per cent sorbitol solution given via the gastric tube, so emptying the small bowel of its contents of drugs and preventing further absorption.

Increase in rate of drug elimination

1 *Diuresis*

In the absence of renal impairment, the patient's kidneys provide a better dialysing membrane than any artificial kidney for the elimination of a drug. However, because renal impairment may have been present before the drug ingestion, or a state of profound hypo-tension might have induced acute tubular necrosis, the ability of the kidneys to excrete a fluid load should be assessed before attempting to force a diuresis. This may be done by administering intravenously a small volume of 10 or 20 per cent mannitol and observing the urinary output during the next few minutes. If there is a significant increase in urine output, it is reasonable to proceed with provoking a diuresis. If not, then intravenous infusion of fluids may precipitate left ventricular failure and pulmonary oedema; in that case other methods of drug elimination must be considered.

When a diuresis is to be produced, two factors must be consid-ered, namely its volume and the urinary pH. The relative import-ance of these factors differs according to the drug under considera-tion. When the reabsorption of the drug across the renal tubular membrane from the lumen of the tubule into the blood stream is not markedly pH dependent, then the only way to modify the rate of excretion is to increase the volume of urine and hence the rate at which it passes through the tubule. This minimises the time during which reabsorption of the drug may occur.

In the case of weak acids, such as salicyclic acid, acetylsalicylic acid, and phenobarbitone, and weak bases such as pethidine, morphine, chlorpromazine, amphetamine, ephedrine, the tricyclic antidepressants and tranylcypromine, alteration of the urinary pH may markedly influence the rate of excretion. The excretion of weakly acidic drugs is increased if the urine is made alkaline, usually by intravenous administration of 1/6 molar lactate solution. Conversely excretion of drugs which are weakly basic is increased if the urine is made more acid by oral or intravenous administration of ammonium chloride.

The intravenous administration of sufficient volumes of fluid, either dextrose or saline, may be enough to provoke and maintain an adequate diuresis, but it is common practice to use a diuretic agent as well, either an osmotic diuretic such as intravenous mannitol (for example 100 ml of 10 per cent mannitol diluted in 500 ml normal saline in one hour), or a diuretic which blocks sodium reabsorption such as frusemide 40–60 mg.

2 *Dialysis*
Peritoneal or haemodialysis should be considered in order to increase the rate of elimination of a drug when blood levels are very high and the clinical condition is poor, or where renal insufficiency precludes the use of forced diuresis.

Care of the unconscious patient

Routine care of the unconscious patient should be scrupulously observed, with particular reference to the skin, with: two-hourly turning and use of a ripple bed if the patient remains unconscious for more than twelve hours; the bladder, with catheterisation under strict aseptic conditions; the bowels, with attention paid to evacuation; and hygiene of the mouth, nose and eyes. The nutritional state must also be observed, with institution of parenteral feeding if necessary.

Psychiatric assessment and treatment

During the recovery phase, the patient may become agitated, distressed or even violent, and may require sedation. If suicidal intent was originally suspected a full psychiatric assessment should be carried out after recovery.

Specific measures

In certain cases of poisoning with centrally acting drugs, additional specific measures may be indicated: narcotic antagonists, such as naloxone or nalorphine, may be used in patients poisoned with morphine, heroin or pethidine, in order to reduce respiratory depression. However, an acute abstinence syndrome may be precipitated if physical dependence has developed on the narcotic drug. Naloxone is superior because it lacks the partial agonist properties of nalorphine and does not itself produce narcotic effects.

Self-poisoning with monoamine reuptake inhibitor antidepressant drugs has become frequent. It produces hypotension, cardiac dysrhythmias and central nervous depression which may be preceded by excitation and convulsions. Management of the cardiac effects has already been discussed. The central effects appear to be associated with the anticholinergic properties of these drugs, and intravenous physostigmine, which crosses the blood-brain barrier may improve the level of consciousness. However, it may itself cause convulsions, bradycardia, and increased salivary and bronchial secretions and should only be used when indicated by the depth of respiratory depression or severity of cardiac dysrhythmias. There is no close relationship between plasma drug level and severity of these adverse effects, and each case must, therefore, be managed individually according to the clinical state.

Over-dosage of monoamine oxidase inhibitors may be associated with hyperpyrexia, for which chlorpromazine is the treatment of choice. If marked hypertension is present, this should be treated with an alpha-adrenergic receptor-blocking drug, such as phentolamine or thymoxamine.

Paracetamol is a relatively safe drug when taken in therapeutic doses, but when taken in excess may cause dose-dependent hepatic necrosis. This hepatotoxicity appears to be due to a toxic metabolite of paracetamol rather than to the parent compound. The best way of managing patients who have taken such a dose of paracetamol is still under investigation, but the following has recently been suggested:

(a) carry out standard procedures for any suspected overdose, as already discussed.

(b) if more than 4 hours and less than 10 hours have elapsed since ingestion of paracetamol, a sample of blood should be assayed for paracetamol content and oral methionine 2·5 g should be given.

(c) The plasma paracetamol level should be plotted on a graph and its position noted relative to a line drawn between 200 mcg/ml at 4 hours and 70 mcg/ml at 10 hours. If the plasma level falls well below the line, significant hepatotoxicity is unlikely.

(d) If the plasma level falls on or above the line, then toxicity is possible, the risk increasing the further above the line the level lies. Such patients should be given intravenous cysteamine up to a total of 3·6 g cysteamine base over the next 20 hours, or oral methionine 2·5 g every 4 hours up to a total of 10 g, provided the administration can commence within 10 hours of ingestion of the overdose. These measures appear to be ineffective after that time.

(e) In addition to such specific measures, appropriate supportive therapy should include fluid replacement with 5 per cent dextrose, vitamin K for prolonged prothrombin time, and maintenance of electrolyte balance.

Suggestions for further reading

BRITISH MEDICAL JOURNAL (Editorial), 'Activated charcoal rediscovered', *British Medical Journal*, vol. 3, 1972, p. 487.

BRITISH MEDICAL JOURNAL (Editorial), 'First aid for poisoning', *British Medical Journal*, vol. 1, 1974, p. 130.

DRIESBACH, R. H., *Handbook of Poisoning*, 7th edn, Blackwell, Oxford, 1971.

GLEASON, M. N., GOSSELIN, R. E., HODGE, H. C., and SMITH, R. P., *Clinical Toxicology of Commercial Products, Acute Poisoning*, 3rd edn, Williams & Wilkins, Baltimore, 1969.

MATTHEW, H., and LAWSON, A. A. H., *Treatment of Common Acute Poisonings*, 2nd edn, Livingstone, Edinburgh, 1970.

MORRELLI, H. F., 'Rational therapy of drug overdose', in *Clinical Pharmacology*, ed. K. L. Melmon, and H. F. Morrelli, Macmillan, New York, 1972, p. 605.

SYMPOSIUM ON PARACETAMOL AND THE LIVER, *Journal of International Medical Research*, vol. 4, Supplement 4, 1976.

WOOD, C. A., BROWN, J. R., COLEMAN, J. H., and EVANS, W. E., 'Management of tricyclic antidepressant toxicides', *Diseases of the Nervous System*, vol. 37, 1976, pp. 459–61.

Subject index

(For individual drugs see index of drug names)

Acetaldehyde, 177, 178
Acetaldehyde dehydrogenase, 177
Acetylation, 39
Acetylcholine, 10–22, 89, 96, 170, 194, 231
Acetylcholinesterase, 21, 170
N-acetyltransferase, 39
Addiction *see* Drug dependence
Adenosine triphosphate (ATP), 19
S-adenosylmethionine, 19, 91
Adenylcyclase, 23, 125, 132
Adrenal medulla, 19
Adrenaline, 9, 11, 23, 29, 43, 44, 127, 157
Adrenergic receptors: adrenergic neurone blocking drugs, 44, 45, 130; alpha-receptor blockers, 22; alpha-receptors, 22; beta-receptor blockers, 157; beta-receptors, 22
Adrenocorticotrophic hormone (ACTH), 150
Affective disorders, 75, 120–48; biochemical basis, 122–4; prophylaxis, 139; treatment, 133–9; *see also* Depressive illness, Depressive reaction, Mania
AFFT *see* Auditory flutter-fusion threshold
Aggresive outbursts in children, 240
Agoraphobia, 160
Akathisia, 106
Alcohol, 43, 45, 51, 81, 82, 98, 99, 157, 167
Alcoholic polyneuropathy, 180

Alcoholism, 174, 176–80
Alkaline diuresis, 40; in treatment of drug overdose, 247–8
Alpha-methylnoradrenaline, 26
Alpha-methylparatyrosine, 95
Alzheimer's disease *see* Presenile dementia
Amphetamine psychosis, 184, 219
Amygdala, 150, 153
Anaesthetics, 43, 99
Analeptic drugs, 243
Analgesic drugs, 99, 232–7
Analgesic tests, 49
Analogue scale, 58
Androgens, 209
Angiotensin, 232
Animal tests, 48–50
Anorectic drugs, 41, 218–22
Anorexia nervosa, 109, 226–7
Anti-androgens, 210
Anti-cholinergic drugs, 37, 42, 44, 127, 241
Anti-coagulants, 45, 155
Anti-depressant drugs, 5, 6, 7, 30, 39, 126–31, 133–7; *see also* Monoamine reuptake inhibiting drugs
Antidiuretic hormone, 133
Antiemetic drugs, 96, 113
Antihistamine drugs, 16, 32, 44, 45, 81, 97
Anti-muscarinic agents, 11; *see also* Acetylcholine
Antipyrine, 42
Anxiety, 6, 7, 23, 25, 48, 68, 74, 149–65; anxiety state, 159, 179,

206; appetite, 224; clinical trials, 68; pain, 229, 236; panic attacks, 159; phobias, 160–1; placebo, 77; psychophysiology, 149–52; rating scales, 58, 68; sexual problems, 205–8; situational anxiety, 160–1; treatment, 157–61

Anxiolytic-sedative drugs: anxiety, 152–61; child psychiatry, 240; classification, 7; critical flicker frequency, 51; depression, 133, 135; driving, 80–2; drug dependence, 180; patterns of psychotropic drug prescribing, 71–4; pharmacology, 152–7; sexual disorders, 208

Aphrodisiacs, 208

Appetite, 214–37; disorders, 223–7; pharmacology, 218–23; physiology, 214–18; psychological factors, 214

Appetite-stimulating drugs, 222–3

Appetite suppressants see Anorectic drugs

Argentophil plaques, 169

Arousal, 90, 149

Arteriosclerotic dementia, 169

Ascending reticular system, 11

Aspartic acid, 16

Ataxia, 94

ATP see Adenosine triphosphate

Atropine-type psychosis, 99

Auditory flutter-fusion threshold (AFFT), 52

Auditory function tests, 52

Auditory hallucinations, 91

Autistic behaviour, 238

Autonomic responses: in anxiety, 151; measurement of, 59–60

Auto-radiography, 49

Aversion therapy, 213

Ball bearing test, 54

Barbiturates, 7, 36, 40, 45; anxiety, 158–60; behaviour therapy, 160–1; dependence, 155, 180–1, 183–4; enzyme induction, 45, 155; pharmacology, 154–5;

phenothiazines, interaction with, 98; poisoning, 155, 245, 246, 248; schizophrenia, 101; sleep, 193, 195–6, 198, 200; withdrawal symptoms, 195–6

Basal ganglia, 13, 14, 27

Beck Depression Scale, 57

Behaviour disturbance in children, 238–40

Behaviour therapy: anxiety, 160; sexual problems, 213

Behavioural tests, 49

Benzodiazepine drugs: anxiety, 152–4, 158, 159, 161; classification, 7; delirium tremens, 167–8, 176–7; depressive reactions, 136–7; insomnia, 198; personality disorder, 175; pharmacology, 32, 152–4; school refusal, 240; sexual problems, 212

Benzoquinolizine, 115

Beta-adrenergic receptor blocking drugs: anxiety, 152, 153; impotence, 210; mechanism of action, 22–3

Biguanides, 221, 225, 226

Bile drug excretion see Enterohepatic circulation

Biological availability of drugs, 65–6

Bipolar depression, 120, 123

Body weight, 109, 214

BOL 148 see 2-bromolysergic acid diethylamide

Bradykinin, 52, 232

Brain stem, 12, 13, 14, 15, 17, 32

Brief Psychiatric Rating Scale, 56

2-bromolysergic acid diethylamide, 15

Bulk agents, 222, 225

Butyrophenones: classification, 7; extrapyramidal symptoms, 99; mania, 137; neuroleptoanalgesia, 234; pharamacology, 32, 93, 99; pupillometry, 63; schizophrenia, 99, 101, 115

Calcium, 20, 124

Cannabis, 4, 8, 180, 181, 185–6, 209

Cardiac dysrhythmia: phenothiazine induced, 108; tricyclic induced, 134
Catatonia, 92, 93
Catecholamines, 23, 29; in anxiety, 151; see also Adrenaline, Dopamine, Noradrenaline
Catechol-O-methyltransferase, 19, 131
Category scales, 58
Caudate nucleus, 13
Central stimulant drugs, 130–1
Cerebellum, 11
Cerebral amines, 11–33
Cerebral arteriosclerosis, 167
Cerebral cortex, 10, 11, 13, 15, 16, 17, 32, 150, 153, 156
CFF see Critical flicker frequency
Chemoceptor, 232
Child psychiatry 238–44
Cholecystokinin, 217
Choline, 20
Choline acetyltransferase, 178
Choline esterase, 124
Cholinergic neurones, 11, 21–2, 124
Cholinergic receptors, 21, 22
Choreoathetosis, 94
Clinical rating scales, 56
Clinical trials, 63–70; controlled, 64–70; double blind, 65–6; matching of patients, 67–8; pilot, 64; randomisation, 66–7; statistical analyses, 68–9
Cognitive function see Intelligence tests
COMT see Catechol-O-methyltransferase
Conditioning see Behavioural tests
Confabulation, 171
Confusional state, 14, 166–7
Consciousness, 192
Continuous sedation, 199
Convulsant activity, 109, 246
Co-ordination, tests of, 48, 53–5
Corticosteroids: barbiturates, interaction with, 45, 155; in affective disorder, 125
Corticotrophin, 125

Cortisol see Corticotrophin
Coumarin anticoagulants: interaction with barbiturates, 45, 155
Creutzfeld-Jacob's disease see Presenile dementia
Critical flicker frequency, 51
Cushing's syndrome, 125
Cyclic AMP: adrenergic receptors, 23; affective disorder, 132; chronic administration of MARIs, 127; endocrine function, 125; receptor blockade, 33; role of phosphodiesterase inhibition, 131
Cysteic acid, 16

D-receptor, 23
Decarboxylase, 27
Delirium see Confusional state
Delirium tremens, 167–8, 177
Delusions: amphetamine induced, 184; depression, 121; l-dopa induced, 14; schizophrenia, 94
Dementia: 168–71; arteriosclerotic, 169; presenile, 168; senile, 169
Demethyltryptamine, 90, 91
Depression: classification, 120; drug induced, 14, 28, 94; rating, 57, 58; treatment, 133–7; see also Depressive illness, Depressive reaction
Depressive illness, 120–6, 134–6; biochemical basis, 122–5; endocrine function, 125–6; prophylaxis, 139–40; psychopathology, 121; treatment, 133–9
Depression rating scales, 57–8
Depressive reaction, 120–1; treatment, 136–7
Diamorphine see Opiate drugs
Dibenzazepine drugs see Tricyclic antidepressants
Dibenzobicyclo-octadienes, 164
3,4-dihydroxymandelic acid, 20
Dibenzocycloheptenes, 116
Dihydroxyphenylalanine (dopa), 13, 25, 26, 29, 129, 194
Diphenylamines, 156

Diphenylbutylpiperidine compounds: anxiety, 156; classification, 7; pharmacology, 99–100; schizophrenia, 99, 102, 105
Diphenylmethanes, 163
Disc dotting test, 54
Disorientation, 166
Diuretics, 46
Doctor-patient relationship, 76
Dopa see Dihydroxyphenylalanine
Dopa-decarboxylase, 13, 25, 26
Dopamine (DA): in biochemical basis of affective disorder, 122; in central nervous system transmission, 11, 13, 14, 18, 19, 21, 23, 24, 25, 27, 28, 29, 30, 31; in drug treatment of depression, 128–30; in pharmacology of neuroleptics, 94–100; in schizophrenia, 88–90
Dopamine receptors, 14, 95
Double-blind technique, 65
Dream sleep, 192
Driving, 80–2, 195
Drug acceptors, 21
Drug costs, 71
Drug defaulting, 74–75
Drug dependence, 180–90; amphetamines, 184–5; barbiturates, 183–4; cannabis, 185–6; cocaine, 185; hallucinogens, 186; opiates, 186–9
Dyskinesia, 14, 107, 108, 113
Dysmnesic syndrome (Korsakoff's psychosis), 166, 171–2, 179–80

ECT see Electroconvulsive therapy
EEG see Electroencephalogram
Ejaculatory disorders, 109, 211
Electroconvulsive therapy, 121, 131, 133
Electroencephalogram: methods of studying behavioural effects of drugs, 50, 61; sleep, 192
Electrolytes, in depressive illness, 124
Electromyography, 64
Electroneurophysiological tests, 50
Endogenous depression see

Depressive illness
Enkephalin, 233
Entero-hepatic circulation, 40
Enuresis see Nocturnal enuresis
Enzyme induction, 42, 155
Epilepsy, 238
Evoked potentials, 62
Excretion, of drugs, 39–40
Extrapyramidal symptoms: butyrophenones, 99; classification, 106–7; phenothiazines, 96; reserpine, 94; treatment, 107–8
Eysenck Personality Inventory, 58

Facilitation, 21
False transmitter, 25, 26
Feeding behaviour, 63, 215
Feeding centres, 215
Fluorescent histochemical techniques, 12
Formication, 185
Frigidity, 160, 203, 209, 212

GABA see Gamma-aminobutyric acid
Galactorrhoea, 97
Gamma-aminobutyric acid, 11, 17, 96, 151, 172, 194
Gamma-glutamyltranspeptidase, 42
Gastric emptying, 37, 41
Gastric lavage, 247
Gate-control theory of pain, 230
Gilles de la Tourette's syndrome, 240
Glaucoma, 134
Glucagon, 221
Glucostatic theory of appetite, 216
Glucaric acid, 42
l-glutamic acid, 11, 16
Glycine, 17
Gustatory hallucinations, 91
Gut motility, 37
Gynaecomastia, 97

H_1 receptor see Histamine
Hallucinations: amphetamine induced, 184; levodopa induced, 14; schizophrenia, 71

Hallucinogenic drugs, 90, 181, 186
Hamilton Anxiety Scale, 56
Hamilton Depression Scale, 57
Hand steadiness, 55
Harmala alkaloids, 30
Hashish *see* Cannabis
Hearing, 52
Heart rate, measurement of, 59
Hebephrenic schizophrenia, 93
Hepatic enzyme induction, 37, 42
Heroin *see* Opiate drugs
5-HIAA *see* 5-hydroxyindolacetic
  acid
Hippocampus, 15, 150, 153
Histamine: central nervous system
  transmission, 11, 16, 25, 27, 30;
  H_1 and H_2 receptors, 16; role in
  pain, 231
Histidine, 16, 27
Histidine decarboxylase, 27
Homocysteic acid, 16
Homovanillic acid, 20
Huntington's chorea *see* Presenile
  dementia
Hydrazine derivatives, 30, 129, 143
17-hydroxycorticosteroids, 150
6-β-hydroxycortisol, 42
5-hydroxyindole acetic acid, 20, 123
5-hydroxyindolylaldehyde, 20
Hydroxylation, 39, 128
p-hydroxy-norephedrine, 26, 29
5-hydroxytryptamine (5-HT): in
  affective disorder, 122-5, 128;
  in anxiety, 151; in central nervous system transmission, 11-31;
  in regulation of food intake, 215,
  220-3; role in pain, 231; in
  schizophrenia, 90; in sexual
  problems, 205; in sleep disturbance, 194
5-hydroxytryptamine antagonists,
  15
5-hydroxytryptamine receptor, 23,
  24
5-hydroxytryptophan, 27
Hyoscine, 11
Hyperkinetic syndrome, 238, 239
Hyperprolactinaemia, 205, 209,
  212

Hypersensitivity reactions, due to
  neuroleptics, 110
Hypertensive reactions, due to
  MAOI therapy, 136
Hyperthyroidism, 218
Hypotension, 101, 103
Hypnotics: benzodiazepines, 153;
  interaction with others drugs,
  43, 45; respiratory depression,
  245
Hypnotism, 193
Hypoglycaemia, 168
Hypothalamic-pituitary pathway,
  14
Hypothalamus: 5-HT concentration, 14; MAO concentration,
  19; NA concentration, 12;
  pathogenesis of anxiety, 150;
  regulation of food intake, 214,
  223; substance P concentration,
  18

Ideas of reference, 92
Implosion, in behaviour therapy,
  160
Impotence: drug induced, 109,
  210-11; pathogenesis, 206;
  treatment, 208-10
Incongruity of affect, 92
Indole derivatives, 93, 114
Insecticides, 42
Insomnia, 196-9
Institute of Personality and Ability
  Testing (IPAT) rating scale, 57
Insulin: appetite stimulation, 222;
  regulation of food intake, 216;
  treatment of anorexia nervosa,
  226-7
Intelligence tests, 55-6
Involutional melancholia *see*
  Depressive illness
Isoprenaline, 29

Jaundice, 103, 110

Kidney, effects of lithium therapy
  on, 132-3
Korsakoff's psychosis *see*
  Dysmnesic syndrome

Lactation, 109
Lateralisation, 55
Latin square, 67
Leukopenia, 110
Light-sensitive dermatoses, 110
Limbic system, 32, 150
Lithium, in the treatment of affective disorders: depression, 136; mania, 137–8
Long-term medication, in schizophrenia, 103–4

M receptor, 23–4
Magnesium see Electrolytes in depressive illness
Major tranquillizers see Neuroleptic drugs
Malonylurea, 6
Mammillary bodies, 171
Mania: biochemical basis, 15, 31, 122–4; clinical picture, 121; prophylaxis, 139–40; treatment, 137–9
MAO see Monoamine oxidase
MARI antidepressants see Monoamine reuptake inhibitors
Marihuana see Cannabis
Matching of patients, 67
Mechanism of drug action, 24; depletion of transmitter, 27–9; increased precursor load, 27; inhibition of transmitter release, 28; inhibition of transmitter synthesis, 25–6; monoamine oxidase inhibition, 30; production of false transmitter, 26; receptor blockade, 31–2; receptor stimulation, 31; release of transmitter, 28–9; uptake inhibition, 30–1
Medulla, 15
Melancholia see Depressive illness
Melanin see Pigmentation
Mescaline, 4, 186
Mesolimbic system, 14, 89, 96
Metabolic effects, of phenothiazines, 109
Metabolic rate, and food intake, 217

Metabolism, of psychotropic drugs: acetylation, 39; conjugation, 39; first pass phenomenon, 38; hydroxylation, 39; liver metabolism, 38; protein binding, 39; steady state blood level, 39; tissue distribution, 39
Methionine, 90
Methionine enkephalin, 233
3-methoxy-4-hydroxy mandelic acid, 20, 124
3-methoxytryptamine, 20
3-methoxy-4-hydroxy–phenylglycol (MHPG), 123
Methyl acceptors, 90
5-methyltetrahydrofolic acid (MTHF), 90, 91
5-methoxy–N, N–diemethyltryptamine (OMB), 90
Methylxanthines, 131
Microinjection techniques, 13
Mill Hill Vocabulary Test, 56
Monoamine hypothesis, of affective disorder, 122–4
Monoamine oxidase: effects of inhibition, 30–1; effects of iproniazid on, 5, 122; effects of reserpine depletion on, 27; location of in gut and liver, 37, 42
Monoamine oxidase inhibitors (MAOIs): classification, 7; depression, 5, 128–30, 136, 143; interaction with other drugs, 129–30, 225, 143; pharmacology, 30, 32, 122, 128–30; phobias, 161; poisoning, 249; sexual effect, 211; sleep disturbance, 194
Monoamine reuptake inhibiting drugs (MARIs): anticholinergic effects, 127, 134; cardiotoxicity, 134, 140; classification, 7, 126, 134; depression, 126–8, 133–6; historical aspects, 5–6; interaction with other drugs, 127, 134; nocturnal enuresis, 241–2; pharmacology, 126–8; poisoning, 249; sexual effects, 211; side effects, 134–6

Mood, 68, 120
Morbid anxiety inventory, 57
Morphine see Opiate drugs
Motor function tests, 53
Motor behaviour, 92
MTHF see 5-methyltetrahydro-
folic acid
Multichannel micropipettes, 50
Multivariate statistics, 69
Muricidal activity test, 49
Muscarine, 9, 21
Muscle ischaemia test, 52
Muscle relaxants, interaction with
beta-adrenoceptor blocking
drugs, 45

Narcolepsy, 199, 219
Narcotic analgesics, 43, 45, 99, 130
Narcotic antagonists, 189, 249
Nepenthe, 3
Neurochemical transmitters, 9–21;
depletion, 27–8; false transmitter synthesis, 25–6; inhibition of release, 28–9; inhibition
of synthesis, 25–6; metabolism,
19–20; see also Acetylcholine,
Dopamine, Histamine, 5-hy-
droxytryptamine, Gamma-
aminobutyric acid, Noradrenaline, Prostaglandins, Substance P
Neuroleptanalgesia, 229, 234
Neuroleptic drugs: anorexia nervosa, 227; anxiety, 156; children,
239–40; classification, 7, 111–13;
confusional states, 167; definition, 7; depression, 136; mania,
131, 137; neuroleptoanalgesia,
234, 236; pharmacology, 93–100,
227; schizophrenia, 100–6; unwanted effects, 106–10
Neurotic depression, 136
Neuroticism, 174
Nicotinamide, 90
Nicotine, 22
Nociceptors, 231
Nocturnal enuresis, 241
Non-compliance see Drug defaulting
Noradrenaline: in anxiety, 150,
157; in appetite and food intake,
215, 219–21; in biochemical
theories of affective disorder,
122–3, 127–30; in biochemical
theories of schizophrenia, 88, 99;
in blockade of neuronal uptake,
43–4; in central nervous system
transmission, 11–32; in sleep
disturbance, 194
Norepinephrine see Noradrenaline
Normetadrenaline, 20
Nurses Observation for In-patient
Evaluation Scale (NOSIE), 56

Obesity, 219, 223–6
Obsessional disorder, 175
Octopamine, 27
Oestrogens, 210, 212
Olfactory hallucinations, 91
OMB see 5-methoxy–N, N–diemethyltryptamine
Opiates: dependence, 180–3,
186–9; historical aspects, 3;
sexual effects, 208–9
Opium, 3
Oral contraceptives: interaction
with barbituarates, 45, 125;
psychological effects, 211
Orthodox sleep, 192
Organic psychiatric syndromes,
166–73; acute confusional state,
166–7; delirium tremens, 167–8;
dementia, arteriosclerotic, 169,
presenile, 168, senile, 169; dysmnesic syndrome (Korsakoff's
psychosis), 171
Orthostatic hypotension, due to:
butyrophenones, 99; phenothiazines, 103, 108; tricyclic antidepressants, 134
Overdosage, treatment of, 245–50
Overt behaviour scales, 56

Pain, 229–37; pharmacology,
232–4; psychophysiology, 229–
32, 234–7; tests of, 52–3
Panic attacks, 159–60
Paradoxical sleep, 192
Paranoid delusions, 92, 93

Paranoid psychosis, 88
Parkinsonian symptoms *see* Extra-pyramidal symptoms
Parkinson's disease, 13, 14, 48, 88–9
Passivity feelings, 92
Pattern theory of pain, 230
Penile plethysmography, 60
Perceptual disorders, 91
Pernicious anaemia, 168
Personality disorders, 148–50, 174–6
Personality traits, 174
Pesticides, 42
PGR *see* Psychogalvanic response
Pharmacokinetics, of psychotropic drugs: blood levels, 40–1; distri-bution and protein binding, 37; drug absorption, 35, 37, 41; drug interactions, 41–6; excre-tion, 39–40; metabolism, 38–9
Phenothiazine compounds: ano-rexia nervosa, 227; antiemetic action, 96; anxiety, 156; auto-nomic effects, 108–9; child psychiatry, 240, 243; classifi-cation, 7, 111–13; confusional states, 167; depression, 136; extrapyramidal effects, 106–8; jaundice, 110; leukopenia, 110; mania, 131–2, 137; metabolic effects, 109; neuroleptanalgesia, 233–4; pharmacology, 30–2, 51, 94–9
Phenylalanine, 12, 19, 217
Phenylephrine, 29, 63
Phipps Psychiatric Clinic Be-haviour Chart, 56
Phobias, 160
Phonemes, 91
Phosphodiesterase inhibition, 126, 131
Physical dependence, 180
Pigmentation, 103, 109
Pick's disease *see* Presenile de-mentia
Pilot clinical trial, 64
Piperazines, 95, 112–13
Piperidines, 95, 112

Placebos, 76–7
Platelet, 31
Plethysmography, 60–1, 151
Pons, 13, 15
Postural hypotension *see* Ortho-static hypotension
Potassium, 124
Precursor load, 27
Presenile dementia, 168–70
'Present Psychiatric State' examin-ation, 56
Presynaptic inhibition, 21
Progestogens, 211–12
Progressive matrices, 56
Prolactin, 14, 88, 89, 96, 97
Propanediols, 155, 162–3
Prostaglandins, 17, 18, 232
Prostanoic acid, 17
Prostatism, 134
Protein binding, 37, 39
Pseudo-parkinsonism *see* Extra-pyramidal symptoms
Psychic dependence, 180
Psychodysleptics, 7, 186
Psychogalvanic response, 60, 151
Psychogenic malnutrition *see* Anorexia nervosa
Psychological rating scales, 55–9
Psychopathology: of affective dis-orders, 121; of schizophrenia, 91
Psychopathy, 174
Psychophysiological measures, 59–63; anxiety, 149–52; electro-encephalography, 61–2; electro-myography, 61; heart rate, 59–60; plethysmography, 60–1; pupillometry, 62–3; skin resist-ance, 60
Psychophysiology, of pain, 229
Psychoses *see* Confusional state, Delirium tremens, Dementia, Depressive illness, Mania, Schizophrenia
Psychostimulants, 7, 209
Psychotic depression *see* Depres-sive illness
Psychotomimetic effects, 15
Psychotropic drugs: biological availability, 35–41; classifi-

cation, 7; cost, 71–2; defaulting, 74–5; definition, 3; driving, effects on, 80–2, 195; mechanisms of action, 24–33; poisoning, 245–50; sexual effects, 208–13
Psylocybin, 51
Pupillometry, 62–3
Pursuit rotor, 55

Randomisation, in clinical trials, 66
Rapid eye movement sleep, 192
Rating scales, 55–9; behavioural, 56; clinical, 56–7; cognitive, 55–6; self-rating, 57; in statistical analyses, 68
Rauwolfia alkaloids, 4, 93, 94
Reaction time, 54
Reactive depression, 136
Receptors, 21–4; adrenergic, 22–3; blockade, 31–2; cholinergic, 21–2; dopaminergic, 23–4; 5-hydroxytryptaminergic, 23–4; morphine (M) receptor, 23; pain receptor, 232; stimulation of, 31
Receptor substances, 21, 23
Renshaw cell, 10
Reserpine: in biochemical basis of affective disorder, 122; induced hypothermia, 49; pupillometry, 63; transmitter depletion, 13, 27, 30, 43; in treatment of schizophrenia, 94; sleep, 194; see also Rauwolfia alkaloids
Reticular activating system, 149
Retinal pigmentation, 103, 109
Reverse mirror drawing test, 55
Ribose nucleic acid, 171

Satiety centre, 215
Schizophrenia: biochemical theories, 88–91; catatonic, 93; classification, 93; clinical picture, 91–3; emotional disturbance, 92; hebephrenic, 93; motor behaviour, 92; paranoid, 93; pathogenesis, 87; perceptual disorders, 91; rating scales, 57; simple, 93; thought disorder, 92;

treatment, 100–16, of acute schizophrenia, 100–4, of chronic schizophrenia, 104–6
School refusal, 240–1
Secondary amines, 39, 127
Secondary receptors, 21
Self-poisoning, 245–50
Self-rating scales, 57
Self-stimulation, 150
Senile dementia, 169
Sensory tests, 50–1
Sequential trial, 69
Serotonin see 5-hydroxytryptamine
Sexual deviations, 212–13
Sexual drive, 203–5
Sexual performance: female, 207; male, 206
Sexual problems, 212–13; deviations, 212–13; frigidity, 160, 208, 212; impotence, 160, 208, 212; physiological basis, 203–7; treatment, 160, 208–13
Situational anxiety, 160
Skin potential, 60
Skin reactions, to neuroleptic medication, 110
Skin resistance, 60
Sleep disturbance, 191–202; activated sleep, 192; continuous sedation, 199; dream sleep, 192; effects of drugs on sleep, 193–6; 'hangover' effects, 195; hypnotism, 193; insomnia, 196–9; narcolepsy, 199; nature of sleep, 191; orthodox sleep, 192; paradoxical sleep, 192; rapid eye movement sleep, 192, 194; withdrawal of hypnotics, 195–6
Smell, tests of, 50
Sociopath, 174
Sodium, 125
Sodium chloride, interaction with lithium therapy, 46
Specific desensitisation, 160
Specificity theory of pain, 230
Specific receptors, 21
Spinal cord, 11, 15, 18
Stammering, 243

Statistical analyses, 68
Storage sites, 21
Striatal areas, 13
Stuttering, 243
Substance P, 11, 18
Substantia gelatinosa, 230
Sulphonylureas, interaction with B-adrenoceptor blocking drugs, 45
Surface electrodes, in electromyography, 61
Sympathomimetic amines: adrenergic receptors, 22; classification, 28; interaction with MAOIs, 44, 129–30; interaction with MARIs, 127; treatment of enuresis, 242
Synapses, 9, 10
Synaptic cleft, 20
Synaptic transmission, 9–24
Synaptic vesicles, 18, 27–8
Synergistic interaction, 43
Syphilis, 168
Tactile hallucinations, 91
Tapping speed test, 54
Tardive dyskinesia, 107
Taste, tests of, 50–1
Taurine, 17
Taylor Manifest Anxiety Scale, 57
Temperature, effect on food intake, 217
Temporal lobe epilepsy, 89
Tertiary amines, 39, 127
Tests of drug activity, 48–63; animal, 48–50; behavioural, 49; biochemical, 49; co-ordination, 53–5; electroneurophysiological, 50; psychological, 55–9; psychophysiological, 59–63; rating scales, 55–9; sensory tests, 50–3
Thalamus, 18
Therapeutic community, 111
Therapeutic ratio, 64
Thermal stimuli, 52
Thermostatic theory of appetite, 217–18
Thioxanthenes: classification, 7; in schizophrenia, 93, 99, 114
Thought disorder, 92

Thyroid, effect of lithium on, 132, 138
Thyroid hormones, 125–6, 132
Tics, 243
Tissue distribution, of drugs, 39
Tolerance, 60; amphetamine, 26; definition of, 180
Toxicological studies, 64
Transmitter substances see Neurochemical transmitter
Tricyclic antidepressants: anticholinergic effects, 129, 134; cardiotoxicity, 127, 134; classification, 7, 126, 140–3; depression, 126–8, 133–6; historical aspects, 5–6; interaction with other drugs, 127, 134; nocturnal enuresis, 241–2; pharmacology, 126–8; poisoning, 249; sexual effects, 211; side effects, 134–6
Tryptophan, 20, 27
Tryptophan hydroxylase, 25, 27
Tyramine: classification, 27, 29; interaction with MAOIs, 42, 43, 44; interaction with MARIs, 126, 129
Tyramine pressor effects, 31, 37
Tyrosine, 25
Tyrosine hydroxylase, 25, 95

Unconscious patient, care of, 248
Unipolar depression, 120, 123
Uptake inhibition, 25, 30
Uptake of neurochemical transmitters, 18, 19, 127–8; uptake$_1$, 128; uptake$_2$, 128
Urinary pH, and excretion of drugs, 39–40, 51

Vasopressin, in pain production, 232
Visual Analogue Scale, 53, 63
Visual function tests, 51
Visual hallucinations, 91
Vitamins, 177
VMA see 3-methoxy-4-hydroxymandelic acid
Vomiting centre, 14

Wakefulness, 192
Wechsler Adult Intelligence Scale, 56
Wernicke's encephalopathy, 171, 179
Wines, interaction of MAOIs with, 130
Wing Scale for Schizophrenia, 57, 58
Withdrawal symptoms: alcohol, 176–7; barbituarates, 183–4; opiates, 187–9

Within-subjects trial, 66

Xanthine derivatives, 131

Yeast products, interaction of MAOIs with, 130
Y-maze, 49

Zung Scale, 57

Index of drug names

Proprietary brand names are printed in small capitals.

ABSTEM *see* Calcium carbimide
Acepromazine, 112
Acetophenazine, 113
1-acetylmethadone, 189
Acetylsalicylic acid, 52, 79, 232, 235, 248
ACTOMOL *see* Mebanazine
AKINETON *see* Biperiden
Alcohol, 3, 43, 45, 81, 82, 98, 99, 157, 167, 212
Alpha-methyldopa, 13, 25, 26, 28
Alpha-methylnoradrenaline, 26
Alpha-methylparatyrosine, 25, 95
Alprenolol, 22
Amantadine, 108
Amitriptyline: absorption and metabolism, 37, 39, 40; in affective disorder, 128, 135, 137, 141; blockade of neuronal uptake, 43, 127; child psychiatry, 241, 242
Ammonium chloride, 248
Amobarbital *see* Amylobarbitone
Amphetamine: in affective disorder, 124, 129, 130; anorectic effect, 218–19, 224; central nervous system transmission, 26, 29, 30; classification, 7; critical flicker frequency, 51; dependence, 184–5; driving, 81; enuresis, 242; hyperkinetic syndrome, 239; narcolepsy, 199; psychosis, 88, 92
Amylobarbitone: in anxiety, 154, 159, 162; classification, 7; in schizophrenia, 101; sleep dis-
turbance, 195, 200
ANAFRANIL *see* Clomipramine
Angiotensin, 232
ANQUIL *see* Benperidol
ANTABUSE *see* Disulfiram
APISATE *see* Diethylpropion
Apomorphine: central receptor stimulation, 14, 31; emetic effect, 96; in sexual behaviour, 205
ARTANE *see* Benzhexol
ARVYNOL *see* Ethchlorvynol
Aspirin *see* Acetylsalicylic acid
ATARAX *see* Hydroxyzine
ATIVAN *see* Lorazepam
Atropine: antimuscarinic effects, 11, 22; in treatment of drug withdrawal, 187
AVENTYL *see* Nortryptyline

BANTHINE *see* Methanetheline
Barbiturates *see* Subject index
Barbituric acid *see* Malonylurea
Belladonna alkaloids, 242
Benacytzine, 156, 163
BENADRYL *see* Diphenhydramine
Benperidol, 116, 213
BENVIL *see* Tybamate
BENZEDRINE *see* Amphetamine
Benzhexol, 14, 43, 107, 137
Benzoctamine, 157, 164
Bethanidine, 28, 43, 44, 46, 127, 130, 211
Biperiden, 108
BOL 148 *see* Bromolysergic acid diethylamide
BOLVIDON *see* Mianserin

Bradykinin, 232
Bretylium, 28
BREVITAL *see* Methohexitone
BRIETAL *see* Methohexitone
Bromocriptine, 14, 31, 205, 209, 212
Bromolysergic acid diethylamide, 15
Burimamide, 16
Butaperazine, 113
BUTAZOLIDIN *see* Phenylbutazone
Butobarbital *see* Butobarbitone
Butobarbitone, 200
Butriptyline, 141

Caffeine, 13, 193, 195, 199
Calcium carbimide, 178
CAMCOLIT *see* Lithium carbonate
Cannabis, 4, 8, 180, 181, 185–6, 209
Cantharidin, 210
Carbamazepine, 238
CARBRITAL *see* Carbromal
Carbromal, 207
Carphenazine, 113
CELLEVAC *see* Methylcellulose
CELLUCON *see* Methylcellulose
Chloral hydrate, 170, 199, 200
Chlordiazepoxide: in affective disorders, 135; in alcoholism, 177; in anxiety, 153, 158, 162; child psychiatry, 240, 243; classification, 6, 7; critical flicker frequency, 51; organic psychiatric syndromes, 168
Chlorimipramine *see* Clomipramine
Chlormethiazole: alcohol withdrawal, 168, 171, 177; opiate withdrawal, 187
p-chlorophenylalanine, 25, 26, 130, 210
Chlorpromazine: analgesic effects, 233; anorexia nervosa, 226–7; anxiety, 156, 163; appetite stimulation, 222; auditory function, 52; child psychiatry, 239–40; CNS transmission effects on, 12, 13, 17, 30, 31, 32;

confusional states, 167; depression, 128, 136; mania, 137; pharmacology, 94–9, 128; schizophrenia, 94–8, 101, 102, 106, 111, 222; side effects, 106–7, 108–10, 222; treatment of drug withdrawal, 188; treatment of poisoning, 248–9
Chlorprothixine, 114, 234
Cimetidine, 16
Cinanserin, 15
Clomipramine, 123, 141, 161, 164, 175, 210
Clonidine, 11, 12, 44
Clopenthixol, 114
Clorazepate, 153, 162
Clorgyline, 129
Clozapine, 100, 115
Cocaine, 4, 30, 129, 180, 181, 185
Codeine, 235
CONCORDIN *see* Protriptyline
Cyclandelate, 169
Cyclazocine, 189, 232
CYCLOSPASMOL *see* Cyclandelate
Cyproheptadine, 220, 222, 227
Cyproterone, 61, 210, 213
Cysteamine, 250

DALMANE *see* Flurazepam
DARTALAN *see* Thiopropazate
Debrisoquine, 28, 43, 44, 46, 127
DEPIXOL *see* Flupenthixol decanoate
Desipramine, 39, 43, 127, 140
Dexamphetamine *see* Amphetamine
DEXEDRINE *see* Amphetamine
Diamorphine, 187, 232, 235
Diazepam: anxiety, 153–62; child psychiatry, 241–3; classification, 6, 7; driving, 81; drug withdrawal, use in, 168, 177, 187; pharmacology, 152–4; sensory tests, effects on, 51, 52; sexual function, 212; treatment of poisoning, 246
Dibenzepin, 142
Dibenzyline, 23
DIBOTIN *see* Phenformin

Dichloralphenazone, 170, 199, 201
Diethylpropion, 193, 220, 224, 226
Dihydrocodeine, 235
Dihydroergotoxine, 169
l-dihydroxyphenylalanine   see
   Levodopa
5,6-dihydroxytryptamine, 220
DILANTIN see diphenylhydantoin
DIMERIN see Methyprylone
Dimethylaminopropyl-phenothia-
   zine derivatives, 95
Dimethyltryptophan, 8
Diphenhydramine, 201
Diphenoxylate, 187
Diphenylhydantoin, 164
DISIPAL see Orphenadrine
Disulfiram, 177
l-dopa see Levodopa
DORIDEN see Glutethimide
Dothiepin, 135, 136, 142
Doxepin, 135, 137, 141, 164
DRINAMYL see Amphetamine
Droperidol, 234
DUROMINE see Phentermine
DUVADILAN see Isoxsuprine

ELAVIL see Amitriptyline
ENSIDON see Opipramol
EPANUTIN see Phenytoin
Ephedrine, 29, 37; enuresis, 242;
   mydriatic effect, 63; overdosage
   248
EPILIM see Sodium valproate
EPONTOL see Propanidid
EQUANIL see Meprobamate
ESBATAL see Bethanidine
Ethchlorvynol, 201
Ethinamate, 201
Ethinyloestradiol, 212
Ethynodiol diacetate, 204
EVADYNE see Butriptyline

Fenfluramine, 44, 109, 164, 220,
   225, 226
FENTAZINE see Perphenazine
FLAGYL see Metronidazole
FLUANXOL see Flupenthixol
Flupenthixol, 14, 136
Flupenthixol decanoate, 105, 114

Fluphenazine, 96, 102, 103, 104,
   105
Fluphenazine decanoate, 104, 105
Fluphenazine enanthate, 104, 113
Flurazepam, 153, 195, 198, 200
Fluspirilene, 99, 103, 105, 116
Folic acid, 170
FORTRAL see Pentazocine
FRENACTIL see Benperidol
Frusemide, 248

Glucagon, 221
Glucophage, see Metformin
l-glutamic acid, 11, 16
Glutethimide, 42, 201
Griseofulvin, 155
Guanethidine, 28, 29; impotence,
   211; interaction with MAOIs,
   44, 46, 130; interaction with
   MARIs, 127

HALDOL see Haloperidol
Haloperidol, 7, 12, 32; anxiety,
   156, 163; dementia, 170; hyper-
   kinetic syndrome, 239–40;
   mania, 137; schizophrenia, 99,
   101, 115; sexual effects, 205;
   tics, 243
Harmala alkaloids, 30
HEMINEVRIN see Chlormethiazole
Heptabarbital see Heptabarbitone
Heptabarbitone, 200
Heroin see Diamorphine
Hexamethonium, 37
5HTP see 5-hydroxytryptophan
HYDERGINE see Dihydroergotoxine
Hydrocortisone, 246
Hydroxyamphetamine, 29
5-hydroxytryptophan, 123
Hydroxyzine, 156, 163
Hyoscine, 11, 22, 31

IMAP see Fluspirilene
Imipramine, 5, 7; affective disorders, 122, 127, 130, 135, 140;
   enuresis, 242; pharmacology,
   30–1, 37, 39, 43; pupillometry,
   63
INDERAL see Propranolol

INDOCID *see* Indomethacin
Indomethacin, 235
INSIDON *see* Opipramol
Insulin: in appetite disorders, 222, 226, 227; interaction with β-adrenergic blocking drugs, 45
INTEGRIN *see* Oxypertine
Iprindole, 142
Iproniazid, 30, 122, 143
ISMELIN *see* Guanethidine
Isocarboxazid, 129, 143
Isoniazid, 39
Isoprenaline, 28, 22, 23
Isopropamide, 242
Isoxsuprine, 169

KEMADRIN *see* Procyclidine

Lactate, 248
LARGACTIL *see* Chlorpromazine
LARGON *see* Propiomazine
LENTIZOL *see* Amitriptyline
LEPONEX *see* Clozapine
LETHIDRONE *see* Nalorphine hydrobromide
Levodopa (l-dihydroxyphenylalanine), 14, 48, 107
LIBRIUM *see* Chlordiazepoxide
Lignocaine, 38
LIMBITROL *see* Chlordiazepoxide and amitriptyline
Lithium carbonate, 6; affective disorder, 125, 132, 136–40; pharmacology, 40, 46, 125, 132
LOMOTIL *see* Diphenoxylate
Lorazepam, 153, 162
LSD *see* Lysergic acid diethylamide
LUCOFEN *see* Chlorphentermine
LUDIOMIL *see* Maprotiline
LUMINAL *see* Phenobarbitone
Lysergic acid diethylamide, 4, 7, 15, 23, 26; dependence, 186; in pain perception, 233

MAJEPTIL *see* Thioproperazine
Malonylurea, 6
MANDRAX *see* Methaqualone
Mannitol, 248

Maprotiline, 124, 128, 134, 135, 142
Marihuana, 4
MARPLAN *see* Isocarboxazid
MARSILID *see* Iproniazid
Mazindol, 221, 225
Mebanazine, 143
Medazepam, 153, 162
MEDOMIN *see* Heptabarbitone
MELLERIL *see* Thioridazine
Mephenesin, 155
Meprobamate, 51, 155, 162
Mepyramine, 16
MERITAL *see* Nomifensine
Mescaline, 4, 7, 90, 91
Mesoridazine, 112
Mestranol, 204
Metaraminol, 246
Metformin, 221, 225
Methadone, 187, 188
Methantheline, 242
Methaqualone, 201
METHEDRINE *see* Methylamphetamine
Methionine, 90, 250
Methixene, 107
Methohexitone sodium, 161, 212
Methotrimeprazine, 113
Methoxamine, 28
Methoxypromazine, 112
Methylamphetamine, 184, 242
Methylcellulose, 222, 225
α-methyldopa, 13, 25, 26
α-methylparatyrosine, 25
Methylphenidate: in affective disorder, 130; effect on sleep, 193, 199; hyperkinetic syndrome, 239; in psychotic disorder, 88, 89
Methyprylone, 201
Methysergide, 15, 220
Metiamide, 16
Metiapin, 100, 115
Metoclopramide, 37
Metronidazole, 179
Mianserin, 49, 128, 134, 135, 136, 142
MILTOWN *see* Meprobamate
MODECATE *see* Fluphenazine decanoate

MODITEN *see* Fluphenazine
MODITEN ENANTHATE *see* Fluphenazine enanthate
MOGADON *see* Nitrazepam
Molindone, 100, 115
Moramide, 234
Morphine: analgesic effects, 52, 235, 236; dependence, 181; pharmacology, 4, 23, 38; sexual problems, 209
MOTIVAL *see* Nortriptyline with perphenazine
MYSOLINE *see* Primidone

Naftidrofuryl, 169
Naloxone, 189, 249
NALLINE *see* Nalorphine hydrochloride
Nalorphine hydrobromide, 189
Nalorphine hydrochloride, 189, 249
NARCAN *see* Naloxone
NARDIL *see* Phenelzine
NAVANE *see* Thiothixine
NEMBUTAL *see* Pentobarbitone
Nepenthe, 3
NEULACTIL *see* Pericyazine
Nialamide, 129, 143
NIAMID *see* Nialamide
Nicotinamide, 90
Nicotine, 22
Nicotinic acid, 99, 180
NITOMAN *see* Tetrabenazine
Nitrazepam, 153, 171, 195, 198, 200
NOBRIUM *see* Medazepam
NOCTAN *see* Methyprylone
NOLUDAR *see* Methyprylone
Nomifensine, 127, 135, 137, 143
Noradrenaline, 246
NORPRAMINE *see* Desipramine
Nortriptyline, 39, 43, 135, 141, 242
NORVAL *see* Mianserin
NOTENSIL *see* Acepromazine

Octopamine, 27
Opipramol, 142, 164
Opium, 3, 208
ORAP *see* Pimozide

Orphenadrine, 14, 43, 107, 137
OSPOLOT *see* Sulthiame
Oxazepam, 153, 158, 159, 162
Oxotremorine, 22, 31
Oxprenolol, 22, 159
Oxypertine, 100, 114, 156, 163

Pantothenic acid, 180
Paracetamol, 232, 235, 249
Parachlorophenylalanine, 194, 205
Paraldehyde, 168, 177, 246
PARLODEL *see* Bromocriptine
PARNATE *see* Tranylcypromine
Pemoline, 130
Penfluridol, 100, 105, 116
D-Penicillamine, 109
Pentazocine, 232, 235
Pentobarbital *see* Pentobarbitone
Pentobarbitone, 17, 193, 200
PERIACTIN *see* Cyproheptadine
Pericyazine, 113, 175
Perphenazine, 113, 135
PERTOFRAN *see* Desipramine
Pethidine, 39, 130, 235, 236, 248
PHASAL *see* Lithium carbonate
Phenelzine, 7, 30, 39, 129, 143, 161
Phenformin, 221, 225
Phenmetrazine, 29, 51, 130, 193, 220, 224
Phenobarbital *see* Phenobarbitone
Phenobarbitone, 102, 154, 239, 246, 248
Phenoperidine, 234
Phenoxybenzamine *see* Dibenzyline
Phentanyl, 234
Phentermine, 220, 225, 226
Phentolamine, 22, 249
Phenylalanine, 217
Phenylbutazone, 235
Phenylephrine, 28, 29, 42, 43, 44, 63
Phenytoin, 36, 42, 155, 164, 238, 246
PHYSEPTONE *see* Methadone
Physostigmine, 89, 124, 246, 249
Pimozide, 7, 99, 103, 116, 123, 137, 156, 163, 219
Pindolol, 22

Piperacetazine, 112
Piperazines, 95, 112–13
Piribedil, 14, 31
PLACIDYL see Ethchlorvynol
PONDERAL see Fenfluramine
PONDERAX see Fenfluramine
PRAXILINE see Naftidrofuryl
PRELUDIN see Phenmetrazine
PRESATE see Chlorphentermine
PRIADEL see Lithium carbonate
Primidone, 238
PRO-BANTHINE see Propantheline
Procainamide, 39
Procaine hydrochloride, 170
Prochlorperazine, 112
Procyclidine, 107, 108
PROKETAZINE see Carphenazine
PROLIXIN see Fluphenazine
Promazine, 95, 115
Promethazine, 5, 54, 94, 102
PRONDOL see Iprindole
Propanidid, 161, 212
Propantheline, 242
Propericiazine, 175
Propiomazine, 112
Propranolol, 22, 32; anxiety, 159;
  first pass phenomenon, 38;
  schizophrenia, 106; sexual
  problems, 210; treatment of
  poisoning, 246
PROTHIADEN see Dothiepin
Protriptyline, 124, 127, 134, 135,
  141
Provera, 210
Psylocybin, 7
Pyridoxine, 180

QUAALUDE see Methaqualone
QUIDE see Piperacetazine
Quinalbarbitone, 195, 200

Rauwolfia alkaloids, 4, 93, 94; see
  also Reserpine
REDEPTIN see Fluspiriline
REPOISE see Butaperazine
Reserpine: in biochemical basis of
  affective disorder, 122; induced
  hypothermia, 49; pupillometry,
  63; transmitter depletion, 13,

27, 30, 43; in schizophrenia, 94;
  in sleep, 194
Rifampicin, 42
RITALIN see Methylphenidate

Salicylic acid, 248
SANOREX see Mazindol
Secobarbital see Quinalbarbitone
SECONAL see Quinalbarbitone
SEMAP see Penfluridol
SERAX see Oxazepam
SERENACE see Haloperidol
SERENESIL see Ethchlorvynol
SERENID-D see Oxazepam
SERENTIL see Mesoridazine
SINEQUAN see Doxepin
SODIUM AMYTAL see Amylobarbi-
  tone sodium
Sodium valproate, 108, 172
SOLACEN see Tybamate
SOMNOS see Chloral hydrate
SONERYL see Butobarbitone
Sorbitol, 247
SORDINOL see Clopenthixol
Sotalol, 22, 159
SPARINE see Promazine
STELAZINE see Trifluoperazine
STEMETIL see Prochlorperazine
Stilboestrol, 212
SUAVIT see Benactyzine
SUBSTANCE 'H' see Procaine hydro-
  chloride
Sulthiame, 238
SURMONTIL see Trimipramine

TACITIN see Benzoctamine
TARACTAN see Chlorprothixene
TEGRETOL see Carbamazine
TEMPOSIL see Calcium carbimide
TENTONE see Methoxypromazine
TENUATE see Diethylpropion
TERONAC see Mazindol
Testosterone propionate, 212
Tetrabenazine, 100, 108, 115, 172
Tetrahydrocannabinol (THC), 185
Thalidomide, 38
Theobromine, 131, 193
Theophylline, 131
Thiamine, 168, 172, 179, 180

Thiethylperazine, 113
Thiopentone, 38
Thiopropazate, 108, 113
Thioproperazine, 113
Thioridazine: in dementia, 170, 172; in schizophrenia, 96, 103, 108, 109, 112; in sexual problems, 210
Thiothixene, 7, 114
Thioxanthine compounds, 7, 99, 102, 114
THORAZINE see Chlorpromazine
Thymoxamine, 22, 249
TINDAL see Acetophenazine
TOFRANIL see Imipramine
Tolazoline, 22
TORECAN see Thiethylperazine
TRANXENE see Chlorazepate
Tranylcypromine, 30, 129, 143, 193, 194, 248
TREMONIL see Methixine
Tremorine, 14
Trichlorethyl phosphate, 200
TRICLOFOS see Trichlorethyl phosphate
Trifluoperazine, 102, 103, 112, 156, 163
Trifluperidol, 99, 115

Trifluopromazine, 95, 112
TRILAFON see Perphenazine
Trimipramine, 140
TRIPERIDOL see Trifluperidol
TRIPTAFEN see Perphenazine
TRIPTIL see Protriptyline
TRYPTIZOL see Amitriptyline
L-tryptophan, 20, 27, 136
TUINAL see Quinalbarbitone
Tybamate, 163
Tyramine, 29, 37, 42, 44, 63, 126, 129
TYRIMIDE see Isopropamide

VALIUM see Diazepam
VALMID see Ethinamate
Vasopressin, 232
VERACTIL see Methotrimeprazine
VESPRIN see Trifluopromazine
Viloxazine, 128, 134, 135, 143
VISTARIL see Hydroxyzine
Vitamin K, 250
VIVACTIL see Protriptyline
VIVALAN see Viloxazine

WELLDORM see Dichloralphenazone

Yohimbine, 210